AF567009

PSYCHIATRIC MEDICINE
- A HANDBOOK -

Psychiatric Medicine
- A Handbook -

James L. Mathis, M.D.
Chairman, Department of Psychiatric Medicine
East Carolina University
School of Medicine

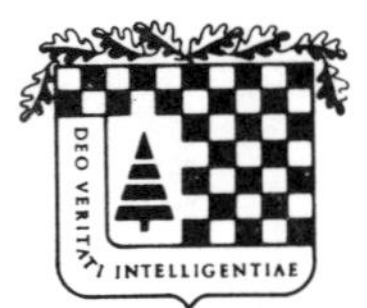

WARREN H. GREEN, INC.
St. Louis, Missouri, U.S.A.

Published by

WARREN H. GREEN, INC.
8356 Olive Boulevard
St. Louis, Missouri 63132, U.S.A.

ISBN No. 0-87527-320-3

Printed in the United States of America

Preface

There are illnesses which are specifically emotional or mental, but all illnesses have emotional components. A young lady with acute Schizophrenia has an obvious mental illness, but what of the mental and emotional aftermath of the high school girl who is paralyzed from the waist down in an automobile accident? How do you relate to the young man with a college scholarship in basketball who loses a hand in a farm machine? The human is a complex organism in which there is a constant interplay among all the parts and, although we must discuss conditions as if they were separate entities, we must strive to understand each person as a dynamic functional unit. A patient with severe coronary artery disease also may have Recurrent Unipolar Depression and neither condition can be treated properly without considering the other one.

This handbook will follow the format and use the terminology of the Diagnostic and Statistical Manual of Mental Disorders of the American Psychiatric Association. Third Edition (DSM III). It will omit many minor and rare syndromes and concentrate on those conditions of clinical importance, but adequate references will be given at the end of each chapter for the reader who desires more theory and definitive details. This will be true particularly of specific treatment aspects, many of which are changing so rapidly that research in neurochemistry and psychopharmacology adds to our knowledge almost daily. A book on psychopharmacology is out of date by the time it reaches the bookshelf.

This book is based on decades of teaching Psychiatric Medicine to students in medicine, dentistry, occupational therapy, nursing, and other allied health disciplines. Jargon will be avoided when possible or, if used, it will be explained in understandable words. The object is to convey to you, in a concise form, useful and practical information which will aid you in your daily work with your fellow humans. The more you know about the aberrations of the human mind, the more you will understand yourself and those with whom you work.

Contents

PSYCHIATRIC MEDICINE
- A HANDBOOK -

I

Development Factors

INFANCY

Medical educators and researchers no longer debate the importance of nature versus nurture. It now is accepted that both play a major role in human development and that they act upon and influence each other. The infant comes into this world with a genetic base which will modify and be modified by, to some degree, every experience that impinges on it. We know that one important factor in determining the form and eventual size of the body is the genetic programming received from the parents, but a 15-year-old boy who is 5'2" tall and weights 115 lbs. will experience the world in a vastly different manner than the same aged youngster who is 6' tall and weights 190 lbs. The size (nature) and the environmental reactions (nurture) will interact to influence the final personality.

A young lady who had recovered from Schizophrenia wrote, "Most people think that what happens to a child before the age of five is not important, but perhaps only those of us who have been mentally ill know that no other time of life is so significant to our futures." She may have exaggerated her point, but much of what she said is true. Those things which impinge upon the child in those years when the billions of brain cells are being formed and interconnected are of utmost importance. Over 90% of brain growth is completed by age six and many basic methods of relating to the world may be indelible.

Personality development can be viewed from several excellent stances. Most of these are modifications of or additions to Freudian concepts. I have chosen a very condensed version of the Freudian theory, but that does not negate the validity of other methods of understanding human growth and development. The important point is to understand that the adult personality is a conglomerate of dynamic forces which interact continuously, but which also go through distinct stages largely determined by biological maturation.

ORAL PHASE

Freud called the first year or so of life the Oral phase. This is primarily a biological term since it specifies the infant's main method of contacting the external world. The infant is dependent totally upon its caretakers and its major method of contact with these caretakers is through the mouth. We have learned since Freud that all bodily contact is of extreme importance and that it is necessary to produce a situation called "bonding" between mother and child. The amount of bodily contact, the way it is given, the manner in which the baby receives nourishment and the situation in which it is given all have much to do with the infant's development of trust in self and others and the development of a sense of security and self-esteem. The baby learns that it can or cannot depend on others to respond to its needs. This can be summarized by saying that there is no substitute for consistently good mothering in infancy to produce a stable, self-assured adult. The phases which follow must be built upon this formulation.

ANAL PHASE

Freud called the second phase of life, roughly from 18 months to three years, the Anal phase. You may prefer to call this the Muscle Training period, because this is a time when the developing human gets control of the muscles of excretion and learns to use the other muscles for locomotion. The child learns much about its ability to control the environment and surmount obstacles and begins to connect its own actions with reward and punishment. The child can receive no greater reward than the approval and the love of the parenting figures and no greater punishment than rejection and neglect. It is unfortunate that in our society many battles develop between parents and child over "potty training," something which should be a perfectly normal function and which separate from the family of origin and to become an independently functioning human being. The end of adolescence arrives, regardless of age, when the youngster has gained emotional independence from the parents and can relate to them as an equal adult.

PSYCHOANALYTICAL THEORY AND THE PERSONALITY

The psychoanalytical terms Id, Ego, and Superego should be understood as theoretical sections of the personality. The psychoanalysts refer to the Id as that basic, animalistic, unsocialized aspect of each of us which says, "I want what I want when I want it!" The young infant is mostly Id, not greatly different from any other young animal. It takes the physical development of the central nervous system and a long and arduous learning process to control this aspect of each of us (that is, to become socialized).

The Ego refers to that part of the personality which assesses and evaluates reality and gives a sense of the self. The child may be attracted to fire and learn that the feeling of warmth at a distance is pleasant, but if he touches the fire, a burned finger is a factor of reality. The child has learned something, and in the future the Ego will tell him that fire can produce discomfort. Ego is rational thinking. It also is that part of each of us that signals self-esteem or the lack of it, and allows us to have a workable security system in relationship to those around us.

The Superego is that internalized sense of values and standards which comes primarily from the relationship with the parent figures and other significant adults. In the beginning, the child will obey the mother when she forbids certain activities, but is apt to obey only so long as the mother is present. As the years advance, especially after six or seven, the child may refrain from doing the forbidden thing even though the mother is not present. The child has internalized the mother's prohibitions as a part of the Superego. Her values and standards (and this may be true of other significant figures in the child's life) have become unconscious parts of the child.

Let us see if we can put these personality aspects in perspective. If you were to see a valuable object which was extremely attractive to you, the Id part of you would say, "Take it." The

Ego part of you might say, "No, do not take it, for if you do so you will be punished in some form and it will not be worth it." Therefore, you might refrain from taking the object because of the reality factors which tell you that the cost will be too great. Since the Superego functions largely outside of awareness, it might be that you saw the object which you so desired, but that you did not think of taking it at all because your Superego forbids you to consider doing such a thing. The mere thought of taking the forbidden object is not in keeping with your internalized sense of values and standards.

Mental illness may involve difficulties in one or more of these theoretical personality facets. For example, there could be such a thing as an uncontrolled Id, and one might have an individual who behaved in a totally selfish, antisocial manner. On the other hand, a defective Ego might result in poor reality testing, as seen in many of the psychoses in which the real world and fantasies are indistinguishable. An overstrict Superego might produce a person who is rigid and inflexible and who constantly fails to succeed up to his perfectionistic standards. A very weak or defective Superego might produce a person who feels little anxiety or guilt and who behaves in self-centered, antisocial ways. These strictly are theoretical concepts, but they aid us in the discussion of personality attributes and human behavior.

The most important aspect of development, assuming a healthy genetic background, is that the child be reared to feel the love and protection of parents from the earliest days. This protection must be balanced by the need of the child to make mistakes, but mistakes which are not fatal and which lead to constructive learning. It is important for the development of future self-esteem for the child to be able to overcome obstacles in a graduated manner. The infant who has absolutely no obstacles to overcome may fail to develop a sense of mastery and self-confidence. On the other hand, the infant whose developmental obstacles are so great that they cannot be overcome may turn out in exactly the same way and lack confidence and a sense of being able to master the environment. In other words, protection that is too extreme so that the child never is allowed to experiment and to make errors may be just as harmful as a total lack of protection and structure in childhood.

No child is reared in utopia. Many anxiety-provoking events will occur and many feelings and attitudes will be overwhelmingly unacceptable. This occurs frequently in childhood and adolescence and, to some degree, throughout life. Many of these unacceptable mental and emotional components will be put out of awareness by a process called repression. Once repressed, they become part of the unconscious mind; totally forgotten, but still present and able to cause or modify behavior. Many of the mental disorders to be discussed are determined largely by unconscious forces. For example, a person with a handwashing compulsion cannot "remember" the cause of this symbolic act of removing guilt, but remains powerless to control it. The forces which make one man an exhibitionist and another unable to tolerate authority are outside of awareness–unconscious. The phobic patient cannot tell you the cause of the irrational fear.

This quick review of developmental factors and their effects on future adjustment does not refer only to the mentally ill patient. These factors make us unique personalities and account for many of those little peculiarities of thought and behavior which attract us to one person or thing and lead us away from others. The desired end result of the process of development is maturity, and one good, simple definition of maturity is "flexibility." The hallmark of immaturity is stereotyped thought and behavior.

BIBLIOGRAPHY

Blos, P.: *On Adolescence.* New York, The Free Press, 1962.

Erikson, E.: *Childhood and Society.* New York, W.W. Norton and Co., Inc., 1950.

Freud, S.: The Ego and the Id. In the Standard Edition of the *Complete Psychological Works of Sigmund Freud.* Vol. 19, London, Hogarth Press, 1961.

Freud, S.: The Sexual Enlightenment of Children. In *Collected Papers,* Vol. 2, pp. 36-44. New York, Basic Books, 1959.

Hartmann, H.: *Essays on Ego Psychology.* New York, International U. Press, 1964.

Klaus, M.H., Jerauld, R., Kreger, N., *et al.*: Maternal attachment: importance of the first post-partum days. *N. Engl. J. Med., 286:*460, 1972.

Lewis, M.: *Clinical Aspects of Child Development,* 2nd Ed. Philadelphia, Lea & Febiger, 1982.

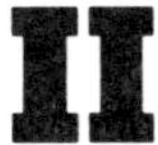

The Role of Stress

An acceptable medical definition for stress is an event or situation which necessitates internal psychological and physiological alterations and/or behavioral changes. This concept implies that any social stimulus or psychological state is capable of upsetting homeostasis and forcing the individual into some form of adaptive behavior. This eliminates the question of whether or not the event or situation is viewed as good or bad, but concerns itself only with the need for an adaptive response by the person. Stress is not necessarily harmful, but whether or not it becomes distress will depend upon:

1. The highly private meaning of the stressful event or situation
2. The capacity of the individual to cope
3. The environmental supports available

The Private Meaning of the Stressful Event

An event which is a catastrophe to one person may be a cause for joy to another. One husband may respond with anxiety and depression upon learning that his wife is pregnant, whereas the same news may be a cause for joy and celebration to another man. Both men would need to adapt to the same situation, but each would do it in an entirely different manner according to the highly specific meaning of the pregnancy to them at that particular time of life.

The private or symbolic meaning of stress is clearly seen in many people who suffer losses or separations. A woman whose father died when she was three years old became very upset when her husband had major, but not unduly dangerous, surgery. Her adverse reaction partially was due to the earlier experience which had sensitized her to separation from the significant male in her life. Long forgotten fears of abandonment were resurrected and experienced as maladaptive anxiety.

The Capacity to Cope

This factor, closely related to emotional maturity and flexibility, is both inherited and learned. It differs remarkably from one person to another and it can be predicted only if one has an accurate history of early life and of how the individual has coped with stressful situations in the past. This will be related generally to early developmental periods and the adaptive skills and self-esteem which do or do not become part of the personality. The more security and love experienced in early years, the more the adult's ability to cope with stress.

Environmental Supports

The most important measurable determinant of an individual's ability to withstand stress appears to be the environmental supports available. Many studies show that this is one of the most significant factors in whether or not one suffers ill effects from stress. When the level of social support is high and readily available, individuals can recover from an amazing amount of stress, but when social support is minimal or absent the ill effects are magnified. Studies have demonstrated the value of the close knit social unit, such as an extended family, as an invaluable defense against the ill effects of stress.

Two other factors are significant when we discuss whether or not stress on the individual plays a role in symptom production. They are:

a. Psychological Specificity
b. Individual Susceptibility

a. Psychological Specificity

This concept refers to the tendency of an individual to

respond to a given stimulus with a reasonably predictable set of reactions. This idea is based upon three factors: stimulus response specificity, individual response specificity, and the current state of the individual.

Stimulus response specificity refers to a situation in which a given stimulus will evoke similar responses in most people. For example, most of us will respond to the immediate threat of an automobile collision with an increased pulse rate, increased respiratory rate, elevated blood pressure, a feeling of profound apprehension, and increased muscle tension. This fear response is specific to the stimulus and will vary only in degree from one person to another.

Individual response specificity means that there are some relatively fixed reactions to stress which will not be general, but which will be a characteristic of a given person. One person may respond to a threat of physical violence by running away. Another may respond by paralysis and inaction, and a third may respond to the threat by counterattacking. The determination of the specific response is many-faceted and includes early learning, genetic predisposition, present situation, and a realistic appraisal of the situation.

The current state of the individual includes such factors as fatigue, the emotional state, the presence of other problems and/or illnesses, and the amount of support immediately available. An exhausted or ill individual will not react the same as if that person were rested and well. The response of a person alone will differ greatly from the reaction of that person when with a familiar group of people.

b. *Individual Susceptibility*

Many studies have demonstrated a correlation between the magnitude of life changes within a given period of time and an individual's susceptibility to some form of illness. These life changes can be viewed as good or bad, but the important factor is how frequently they occur and how much adaptation they require. The studies also show a marked variation among individuals in resistance to all types of stresses. Resistance to stress and illness varies from one person to another, but a variation also exists in a given individual from one time to another. Individual susceptibility is a complex condition relating equally well to all forms of stress from the purely social to the physical.

The Life Change Unit Scale is a method of attaching arbitrary values to events in an individual's life. It uses a baseline of 100 points for the death of a spouse, an event which requires more adaptive response and change than any other one in ordinary living. A definite relationship has been shown between the total Life Change Units an individual amasses over a year and the development of an illness or personal difficulty over the next year. This scale has no individual predictive value but is useful in demonstrating in large groups that the amount of stress which an individual accumulates has a definite effect upon future health.

PERSONALITY TYPES

There is good evidence for an increased susceptibility to coronary artery disease and an increased death rate in men with a Type A behavior pattern. This pattern describes men who are highly competitive, ambitious, goal-oriented, and pressured by time; who react to frustrations with hostility and constantly appear to be striving to meet deadlines. It may be that other personality patterns are equally susceptible to different conditions or that they predispose to a life-style that modifies susceptibility. This may be true of both physical and mental illness.

By what mechanism does stress affect mental, emotional, and physical health? Research has shown a definite correlation between changes in daily living patterns and the levels of cholesterol, uric acid, and cortisol in the blood. The cortisol level may rise as much as 500% following a very stressful event such as a threat to job security. Cholesterol levels rise significantly following anxiety-provoking or worrisome family problems. This fits in with our knowledge that cortisol levels also increase during severe depression. Unresolved stress has been shown to reduce the levels of the reproductive hormones in both males and females. It was noted that most young women placed in World War II concentration camps soon ceased to menstruate, and up to 10% of girls leaving home for college will not menstruate for from one to three months.

What can one do to prevent stress from becoming distress?

It is obvious that one cannot avoid stress, indeed a certain amount of it is essential for a full and rewarding life, but two factors may be useful:

1. Social Supports
2. Anticipatory Guidance

Social Supports

Providing social supports may be one of the best ways of preventing stress from becoming distress. The loner is the one most vulnerable. There is no substitute for the supporting effects of family and friends. Support also can come from organizations such as churches, clubs, and work associations. The old extended family, now rapidly disappearing, was one of the world's best insurances against the ill effects of stress.

Anticipatory Guidance

Anticipatory guidance refers to an active assessment of possible future stresses and the anticipation of methods of dealing with them. This may not be possible in unanticipated stress, but many situations do allow it. Anticipatory guidance can be used on an everyday basis in surgical procedures, separations, some chronic illnesses, and other predictable events. A certain amount of worry is advisable under these circumstances. This "worry work" appears to prepare the individual's defenses for a stressful onslaught so that it does not come as a total surprise. It has been shown that the body's glandular and immune system is able to prepare itself and to withstand stress with fewer complications when this "worry work" occurs under proper control. Caretaking people in medicine may need to help patients facing a known stress to anticipate it realistically and to explore the factors available to alleviate the immediate discomfort and the possible long-term ill effects.

A new type of stress has been recognized in recent years. Its name, existential stress, denotes its pervasive chracter in modern society. It is the background music in all our lives. It is composed of anxieties over nuclear stockpiles, energy depletion, inflation, ecological disasters, overpopulation, and a host of threats to which we cannot respond constructively. We prefer to deny the existence of these conditions, but they do not go away and they influence, like hidden icebergs, our routine lives.

Keep in mind that stress alone does not cause mental, emotional, or physical illness. Stress plays a precipitating role, not a causative one. We frequently look for precipitating events in people with mental or emotional decompensation, but it is dangerous and oversimplified to accept these events as the only factors involved. Each case must be evaluated carefully, with an open mind and one must ask, "Why did this particular event or situation produce this reaction at this time?"

BIBLIOGRAPHY

Caplan, G.: *Principles of Preventive Psychiatry.* New York, Basic Books, 1964.

Friedman, M., and Rosenman, R.: *Type A Behavior and Your Heart.* Greenwich, CT, Fawcett, 1974.

Holmes, T., and Rahe, R.: The Social Readjustment Rating Scale. *J. Psychosom. Res., 11:*213-218, 1967.

Janis, I.: *Psychological Stress.* New York, John Wiley & Sons, 1958.

Lipowski, Z.: Psychosomatic medicine in the seventies: an overview. *Am. J. Psychiatry, 134:*233-244, 1977.

III

The Genesis of Functional Disorders

There are mental and emotional disorders for which no organic etiology can be identified. This does not mean that there is no organic component, and it may be that the use of the word "functional" merely betrays our ignorance of the complex neurochemistry of the brain. Future research may show that there are organic lesions but that they are of a neurochemical or hormonal nature which our present techniques are unable to identify. The word "functional" is almost synonymous with psychological.

The following diagram is a grossly oversimplified summary of the genesis of functional illnesses. It represents an amalgamation of theories, but is based primarily on the concepts of psychoanalysis, however loosely. It is intended only to form a framework for understanding human behavior and the ways in which it is influenced by external and internal stimuli, many of which are beyond conscious control.

The reader is cautioned against accepting this format in toto as proven fact, even though certain parts are scientifically valid. The four modifiers of coping techniques are not questioned by authorities on human behavior, but the items under "Maladjustment" can be debated. Those who believe strongly in learning theory may object to the role assigned to anxiety.

The text to follow the diagram will explain the components in greater detail and define the terms as they are used in Psychiatric Medicine.

A MODEL FOR FUNCTIONAL DISORDERS

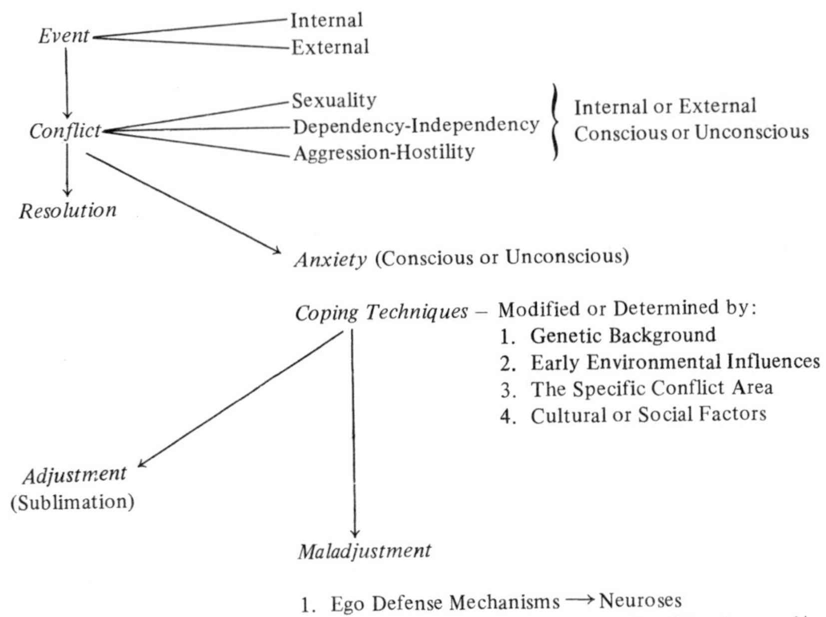

1. Ego Defense Mechanisms → Neuroses
2. Denial and Action → Personality Disorders and/or Minor Affective Disorders
3. Autonomic Nervous System Overaction → Psychophysiological Disorders
4. Decompensation (with or without trial of 1, 2, or 3) → Psychoses

AN EVENT

The event or situation which initiates the development of a Functional Disorder may be an act, impulse, wish, or fantasy, For example, a very religious young lady with strict moral standards finds that she is daydreaming about sexual activity with an attractive male acquaintance. This immediately produces a conflict between her basic human desires and her very strict moral background and she feels guilt and shame. The "event," in this case, is internal. Another person develops an extreme dislike and resentment of an employer. This person has been reared to believe that all feeling of anger and hostility is forbidden and to think that all anger must be suppressed. At some level, this person cannot help feeling the anger is justified even though it is forbidden, therefore a conflict has developed.

THE CONFLICT

Almost all human conflict which leads to intrapsychic difficulty centers around one or more of three areas: sexuality, aggressivity or hostility, and dependency versus independency. These conflicts may be internal or external. An example of an internal conflict is the young lady with the sexual fantasies as noted above. The same is true of the person with the anger and resentment, but this could have been external in origin. Let us assume that the individual feeling the anger has no deeply ingrained inhibitions and does not think that there is anything wrong with this feeling. However, to express the anger openly to the employer would be almost certain to produce a catastrophe in that person's career. A conflict has developed because of the realistic results of expressing the honest emotion.

The predominant area of conflict appears to have changed over the past couple of generations in Western society. Freud and others wrote of the great importance of conflicts involving sexuality and the production of the classical neurotic illnesses. It was extremely important to repress and suppress actions and feelings of sexuality in the period of our history known as "Victorian." This attitude has changed, sexuality has become a very open and acceptable aspect of our living in recent times and it appears that the conflicts surrounding it have decreased accordingly. There has been a corresponding decrease in the classical neuroses seen in psychiatric clinics.

On the other hand, conflicts surrounding hostility and dependency appear to have increased in recent years. Longer and longer periods of education have necessitated an increase in the time a young person is dependent upon parental figures. Young men no longer go directly from childhood into an apprenticeship or to gainful occupation. Aggressive and hostile impulses have become harder and harder to exteriorize in a crowded society where people live in apartment houses and suburban complexes and tend to work in close proximity to each other. Contrast this with the open, agricultural society of a few years ago. Some people feel that the increases in Psychosomatic Disorders and in Personality Disorders reflect the changes in the basic area of conflict.

ANXIETY

The term anxiety is used here to refer to an internalized discomfort, to a drive to act or to move in some way. The term is not used to refer to shakiness, nervousness, or overt fear. This anxiety refers to the internal motivation of behavior and it implies that some change in thinking, feeling, or behavior will occur to alleviate the discomfort.

COPING TECHNIQUES

The individual characteristics and traits which make each of us a unique personality are determined largely by the coping techniques we develop. It is not possible to live without conflict and anxiety, but most of us do not cope in such a manner as to produce maladjustment. A health adjustment to the conflict may occur by resolution or by sublimation.

Resolution means that changes in living, feeling and/or thinking are made so that the conflict no longer exists, therefore the anxiety disappears. Our young lady with the sexual conflict could come to realize and accept that all humans have sexual fantasies and that there is nothing wicked or evil about this. She might learn to relax her overactive inhibition and see herself as a normal human. Our person with the anger and resentment toward the employer might come to see that these feelings were unjustified or, on the contrary, might find it necessary to change job situations. In either event the conflict would dissipate.

Sublimation refers to channeling the impulse, wish, or fantasy into some socially acceptable act that satisfies the original feeling. By this mechanism, a person with intense feelings of anger and hostility may sublimate these feelings by an active sport or by some strenuous labor such as chopping wood.

The factors thought to determine and/or modify coping techniques are:

1. Genetic Background
2. Early Environmental Factors (learning)
3. The Specific Area of Conflict
4. Cultural and Social Factors

Genetic Background

Some portion of our basic personality is inherited. It frequently is not easy to determine the difference between what is inherited and what is learned, but we know that a predisposition to certain types of depression is genetic. We also know that a predisposition to other mental illnesses and to alcoholism have a genetic component. It may be that many of our everyday traits and attributes are equally determined before birth. Every mother of several children can tell you that each of them responded differently from early infancy.

Early Environmental Factors (Learning)

There is much evidence that the genetic substrate of a human being can be modified considerably by environmental factors. The child who must spend part of its early life in an incubator because of prematurity will be denied much of the bodily contact so needed for bonding with the mother. A child raised in a home in which there is chronic conflict between the parents will not know the safety and security needed for the development of trust and self-esteem. The overprotected child may respond the same as the very neglected one and become an adult deficient in self-reliance and self-confidence. There is much evidence that the child who suffers physical abuse in childhood becomes the abusing parent in later life. This trait may be more learned than genetic.

It is probable that we learn mechanisms, called Ego Defense Mechanisms, to defend ourselves against anxiety. A child reared in a family where a parent responds to all conflict by developing physical symptoms may have headaches under tension. A child reared by parents who continually blame someone else for everything that goes wrong may grow up to be one who blames others for its deficiencies and mistakes and who seldom accepts responsibility for its own frailties.

Specific Area of Conflict

The area of the conflict may determine to some degree the coping mechanism used. Psychoanalysis teaches that conflicts surrounding sexuality have been associated with the development of the classical neuroses such as phobias, hysterical reactions, and obsessions. Dependency-independency conflicts have been associated with the development of Psychosomatic Disorders such as peptic ulcer and asthma. Conflicts surrounding aggressivity and hostility have been associated with the Personality and Behavioral Disorders and perhaps even with hypertension and cardiac diseases. No one maintains that there is great specificity here, but the possibility must be considered.

Social and Cultural Milieu

The family, the social group, and the culture in which an individual lives exert a powerful influence on all behavior. Certain social groups, such as Orthodox Jews, have strong prohibitions against the abuse of alcohol and alcoholism is rare among these people. Some cultures tolerate tremendous freedom of sexual behavior up to a certain age, and they have been reported to have a decreased amount of sexual problems in adulthood. The incidence of the severe psychoses are not changed by cultural factors, but the manner in which these illnesses become symptomatic is determined largely by the social group and its standards.

MALADJUSTMENT

It must be understood that the following constructs mainly are theoretical and that they aid us only in understanding human behavior. They must not be taken as hard facts, and the interactions and variations are numerous.

Neuroses

The neuroses (Anxiety and Dissociative Disorders) largely stem from the overuse or the misuse of Ego Defense Mechanisms. For example, the overuse of displacement and symbolization can produce a phobia, which is an unreal fear. A person with a cat phobia may be well aware of the fact that the cat is harmless, but the cat has become a symbol of something from the past that was horrifying to that person. That horrifying situation is displaced onto the symbol, the cat, so that the person reacts "as if" the event were occurring when in contact with the symbol.

Obsessive-compulsive Neuroses use the mechanisms of magical thinking and of atonement. Ritualization also plays a part in that the person may atone for some imaginary wrong by a complicated ritual which has no realistic meaning, but which makes life difficult. Compulsive hand washing is an example.

The many other mechanisms that may be used are of no great practical value or will be discussed under the specific diagnostic categories to which they pertain.

Personality Disorders

The Behavioral and Personality Disorders, including alcoholism, substance abuse of other kinds, and many of the sexual disorders most often stem from the use of denial and acting out. This means that the individual denies, or fails to see or recognize, that anything is wrong. Rather than face the anxiety, this person chooses to act in some manner so as to dissipate the anxiety. Unfortunately, the actions usually are antisocial or self-defeating as seen in the alcoholic who may abuse alcohol whenever the anxiety titer rises. This person will deny that there is anything wrong with this action but, by the very action, the anxiety is temporarily dispersed. Another may commit a crime. The unfortunate fact is that the result is only temporary and the immediate control of the anxiety produces more harm than good.

Psychophysiological Disorders

The Psychophysiological Disorders may arise from a dysfunction of the autonomic nervous system. Most people feel that there is a large genetic predisposition here, but also that some of it may be learned. Overactivity of the vagus nerve may be a part of the production of peptic ulcer. The symptoms of fast heart rate, smothering sensations, sweating, shakiness, etc., due mostly to overactivity of the sympathetic nervous system, are the classical symptoms of Anxiety Disorder.

Psychoses

The Psychoses probably have much larger genetic and biological components and more is known about their chemical aspects. Schizophrenia and Bipolar Depressive Disorder definitely have genetic components and there are specific neurochemical factors involved, but the onset of these conditions may be due to a decompensation of the attempts at coping, and the symptoms of these conditions may be determined by the same factors which modify the coping techniques. We will discuss these conditions in more detail under their specific diagnostic categories.

BIBLIOGRAPHY

Freud, A.: *The Ego and the Mechanisms of Defense.* New York, International U. Press, 1953.

Horney, K.: *Our Inner Conflicts.* New York, W.W. Norton, 1945.

Lader, M., and Marks, I.: *Clinical Anxiety.* New York, Grune & Stratton, 1971.

Mead, M.: *Sex and Temperament in Three Primitive Societies.* New York, William Morrow, 1935.

Yahraes, H.: *Genes and Mental Health.* Science Reports, N.I.M.H., DHEW Publication No. (ADM)78-640, 1978.

IV

Disorders of Infancy and Childhood

This section will not discuss all the disorders of infancy and childhood, but will focus on the three diagnostic categories which occur with sufficient frequency to be clinically important or which are specific to this age range. These disorders are:

1. Mental Retardation
2. Attention Deficit Disorder
3. Infantile Autism

MENTAL RETARDATION

Mental retardation means that the person functions below the average intellectual level and that this results in or is associated with an impairment in adaptive behavior. The onset must have been before the age of 18. The below average intellectual functioning refers to an I.Q. of 70 or below on an expertly administered I.Q. test, usually the WISC (Wechsler Intelligence Scale for Children). Deficiency in adaptive behavior means that the individual fails to meet the levels of social responsibility and personal independence expected of his or her age and cultural group. This judgment calls for a thorough knowledge of the individual, the family, and the social setting. The diagnosis of Mental Retardation has such far-reaching consequences for the child and its family that it must not be made without absolute certainty.

The cause of Mental Retardation may be primarily biological, psychosocial, or an interaction of both. Known chromosomal and metabolic disorders such as Down's syndrome (Mongolism) and Phenylketonuria (a defect in metabolism of phenylalanine) account for about 25% of the cases, but no known biological factor accounts for the disorder in the remaining 75%. There often is a familial pattern of mental retardation in parents and siblings, and the lower socioeconomic classes are overrepresented. Birth trauma, severe malnutrition, psychosocial deprivation, and early maladaptive childrearing experiences have been implicated. Approximately 1% of the population of this country meets the criteria for Mental Retardation at any one time, and the disorder is nearly twice as common among males as females.

Sub-types of Mental Retardation	*I.Q. Levels*
Mild	50-70
Moderate	35-49
Severe	20-34
Profound	Below 20

Mild Mental Retardation

This group accounts for approximately 80% of the mentally retarded. These people are educable in that they may develop social and communication skills which are sufficient to make them indistinguishable from normal children until they reach school age. The first sign of the retardation usually is an inability to learn as fast as their fellow students. These children have the ability to advance academically to approximately the sixth grade level and, with guidance and support, they frequently can achieve social and vocational skills adequate for minimum self-support in adulthood.

Moderate Mental Retardation

This group, approximately 12% of the whole, is considered "trainable." They can learn to talk and to communicate fairly well, but they develop a poor grasp of social skills. Parents usually note them in early childhood as "slow" in all aspects of development. They may profit from vocational training and be able to function at about the second grade level with moderate supervision. They may contribute to their own support as adults by performing unskilled work under close supervision or in sheltered workshop situations, but rarely can they exist alone and support themselves.

Severe Mental Retardation

The severely retarded, approximately 7% of the whole, show evidence of poor motor development and minimal speech achievement at the preschool level. They may be trained in elementary personal hygiene, but generally will be unable to profit from formal vocational training. As adults, they will be able to perform only simple tasks under very close supervision.

Profound Mental Retardation

Only about 1% of the retarded are at the Profound level. These unfortunate children have little potential for sensory motor functioning and will require a highly structured and constantly supervised environment. The possibility of independent functioning at any age is nil and many will be institutionalized for life.

Treatment

All children suspected of being retarded should have a thorough workup by a specialist in the field. Some of the uncommon metabolic conditions can be halted or reversed if detected soon enough. When there is no reversible cause, well organized plans of education and training may make a great difference in the eventual outcome, especially in the first two sub-types. The families of retarded children need much support and guidance since the modern course is to maintain the child in the community when possible. A retarded child always is a tragedy which upsets the entire family and produces emotions ranging through guilt, anger, resentment, and shame.

ATTENTION DEFICIT DISORDER

The essential features are a very short attention span and impulsive behavior. This diagnostic label has replaced the older and less meaningful terms of minimal brain damage, minimal brain dysfunction, minimal cerebral dysfunction, hyperkinetic syndrome, and several other outmoded designations. This condition may occur with or without hyperactivity, although it is not known whether these two forms represent variations of a single disorder or two distinct conditions.

Attention Deficit Disorder with Hyperactivity is characterized by the inability to pay proper attention, impulsivity, and hyperactivity. These children are typically called "brats." They give the impression that they are not listening or that they pay no attention to what is said to them. Their school work characteristically is sloppily performed and they are impulsive in actions and decisions. They cause constant difficulty in the classroom since they have problems sitting still and are apt to be in almost incessant motion. They are particularly troublesome in situations where sustained attention is needed and/or they are expected to work or play cooperatively with others. This means that they may not be so much trouble at home where they can move about at will and play alone.

No cause can be identified for most of these cases, but there is evidence for an inherited factor and for some relationship between this disorder and alcoholism and antisocial behavior in the parents.

The diagnosis frequently is not made until the child begins school and is forced to comply with rules and regulations and sit still for long periods. These children often are stubborn, bossy, tend to be bullies, show quick changes of mood, and have an extremely low tolerance for frustration. The hyperactivity aspect often does not persist past early adolescence, but they may have great emotional problems because their poor work at school and poor relationships with their peers retards their emotional growth and maturation and especially their ability to socialize.

Treatment

Treatment of the hyperactive type of Attention Deficit Disorder is controversial, but most frequently Ritalin (methylphenidate) is used to ameliorate the hyperactivity. This may allow an otherwise uncontrollable child to remain in school and advance normally. Since the drug may decrease growth hormone output, holidays from Ritalin are suggested at vacation times and on weekends. The drug can be stopped periodically to determine whether it is still needed. Most children will be able to discontinue the medication at or before puberty with no return of the hyperactivity. These children do have more emotional problems in adulthood than the average person, but whether this is due to the basic condition or to the turmoil the condition produces in early years is unknown. Probably both factors interact.

Attention Deficit Disorder without Hyperactivity has all the features above except for the hyperactivity. They do not respond well to Ritalin and a very careful and complete workup is needed to exclude brain lesions and specific learning disorders.

INFANTILE AUTISM

The most obvious characteristics of Autism are a lack of responsiveness to other people, severe impairment in communication, and bizarre responses to the environment. These characteristics develop within the first 30 months of life. The etiology has been associated with known organic conditions such as maternal rubella but, in most instances, the cause is unknown. Some authorities believe that the condition represents the earliest form of Schizophrenia, but there is little evidence to support this opinion.

These children fail to cuddle from the earliest days and parents note a lack of eye contact and normal facial responsiveness very quickly. They seem to have a real aversion to affection and physical contact, and often parents think that the child has some difficulty seeing or hearing. They tend to treat the parents and other adults or siblings as if they were mechanical objects and, as they grow older, there is a complete failure to develop cooperative play and friendships. There is some variation in the condition and, occasionally, autistic children may reach the stage where they can become passively involved with other children in simple play roles. The severely autistic children develop no verbal skills and language may be totally absent. Even nonverbal communication such as facial expressions and hand gestures frequently are absent or inappropriate.

Most of these children show a strong attachment to objects in that they may insist upon the same object being present continually. There may be ritualistic behavior such as peculiar hand movements or insisting that all of the objects in their room be in exactly the same place at all times. Some of these children have a fascination with spinning and turning movements.

It is assumed that many of these children have a low I.Q., but this is difficult to measure in an autistic child. Unfortunately, the disorder is chronic, and only about one out of six autistic children may make a minimal social adjustment by adulthood. Infantile Autism is a tragedy with far-reaching effects upon the entire family. There is no specific treatment for Autism, but most areas have clinics which attempt to reach the child through behavioral methods and to help both child and parents to live as normally as possible. Complete recovery from true Autism is very rare.

There are many other conditions of infancy and childhood, but most of them are not specific to that age group and will be discussed in other chapters. Children have Schizophrenia, anxiety reactions, and depression, but if one makes allowances for the age of the patient (an important point) the symptoms are not that different from those seen in adulthood. Conditions such as sleep-walking, bed-wetting (enuresis), lack of bowel control beyond the expected age (encopresis), and conduct disorders are best seen as symptoms of an underlying disturbance rather than as disease entities in themselves. These conditions always require a complete assessment of the child and its family. That also is true of all aberrant behavior. It is dangerous to assume that the child with an obsessive preoccupation at age nine will "outgrow" the condition in a few months. That may be true, but all too frequently some form of the condition will surface again in adolescence or early adulthood, and often in a more serious degree.

BIBLIOGRAPHY

Benda, C.: *Down's Syndrome: Mongolism and its Management.* New York, Grune & Stratton, 1969.

Brady, R.: Inherited metabolic diseases of the nervous system. *Science, 193:*733-739, 1976.

Morrison, J., and Stewart, M.: Evidence for a polygenetic inheritance in the hyperactive child syndrome. *Am. J. Psychiatry, 130:*791-792, 1973.

Ornitz, E., and Ritvo, E.: The syndrome of autism: a critical review. *Am. J. Psychiatry, 133:*609, 1976.

Satterfield, J., Cantwell, D., and Satterfield, B.: Pathophysiology of the hyperactive child syndrome. *Arch. Gen. Psychiatry, 31:*839-845, 1974.

V

Organic Mental Disorders

Organic Mental Disorders are such a mixed group that no single description can characterize them all in detail. The differences in clinical signs and symptoms depend on the localization and the nature of the brain lesion, the mode of onset, the progression, the duration and, to some degree, the previous personality of the individual. The common characteristic of all these disorders is a psychological or behavioral abnormality associated with transient or permanent dysfunction of the brain. All psychological processes, normal and abnormal, depend on brain function, but here we deal with conditions in which an organic factor can be demonstrated or highly suspected. A bullet through the brain is an obvious organic factor producing more or less permanent damage, but an overdose of a toxic drug may produce severe organic symptoms due to deranged brain function of a temporary nature.

Organic Brain Disorders are increasing steadily in medical practice. The number of aged people is rising; more people survive head injuries with damaged brains; alcohol and drug abuse are producing increasing numbers of brain-damaged individuals. More people are surviving heroic surgical procedures and cardiac diseases which, not infrequently, leave some residual brain dysfunction due to temporary brain anoxia.

The signs and symptoms of each category will be outlined, but the general characteristics of all Organic Brain Disorders are:

1. Impairment of orientation including time, place, person and/or situation.
2. Impairment of memory with recent memory usually lost before remote memory is affected.
3. Impairment of the intellect, including attention, concentration, reasoning, and learning.

4. Impairment of judgment, especially when unfamiliar situations arise or abstract thinking is involved.
5. Emotional lability: mood changes from fear to depression and apprehension may occur rapidly.

ORGANIC BRAIN SYNDROMES

1. *Delirium and Dementia,* in which cognitive impairment (thinking) is relatively global.
2. *Amnestic Syndrome and Organic Hallucinosis,* in which relatively selective areas of cognition are impaired.
3. *Organic Delusional Syndrome and Organic Affective Syndrome,* in which there are features resembling schizophrenic or affective (mood) disorders.
4. *Organic Personality Syndrome,* in which the personality primarily is affected.
5. *Intoxication Withdrawal,* in which the disorder is associated with ingestion or reduction in use of a substance ordinarily considered addicting.
6. *Atypical or Mixed Organic Brain Syndromes,* which includes all those not classifiable in one of the other five categories.

Delirium

This refers to a disturbed state of consciousness: that is, a reduction in contact with the environment. These patients have difficulty in holding attention to both internal and external stimuli. They misinterpret sensory input and have a poor ability to think. Usually, there is a disturbance of sleep/waking states and there is some degree of psychomotor hyperactivity. The onset usually is rapid and the symptoms show much fluctuation from one hour to the next.

The delirious person cannot carry on a sensible conversation and usually shows disorientation to time, place, person and/or situation. Visual hallucinations (seeing things that are not there) are common, as are delusions (false beliefs). There are all degrees of Delirium from mild confusion to total disorganization. Most of these patients will be extremely irritable and frightened and they must be protected from injuring themselves and others.

There can be many causes of Delirium. They vary from systematic infections to metabolic disorders, post-operative confusions, substance intoxication, and withdrawal. One of the delirious states most frequently seen by doctors is that due to withdrawal from prolonged use of alcohol (Delirium Tremens).

Diagnostic Criteria for Delirium

A. Clouding of consciousness with reduced capacity to pay normal attention to environmental stimuli.
B. At least two of the following:
   1. perceptual disturbance such as misinterpretations, illusions, or hallucinations
   2. incoherent speech
   3. disturbance of sleep/wakefulness cycle with insomnia or daytime drowsiness
   4. increased or decreased psychomotor activity
C. Disorientation and memory impairment.
D. Clinical features that develop over a short period of time and tend to fluctuate over the course of a day.
E. Evidence from history, physical examination, or laboratory tests of a specific organic factor thought to be the cause of the disturbance.

Dementia

This refers to loss of intellectual functioning of sufficient severity to interfere with social or occupational activities. The defect involves memory, judgment, abstract thought, and other higher brain functions. Changes in personality and behavior are common. Delirium and Dementia may coexist but, if the diagnostic points listed above for Delirium are present, that diagnosis should be considered first. Memory impairment is the symptom seen most frequently and varies from mild forgetfulness to complete absence of memory.

Impairment in abstract thinking becomes evident when the patient must cope with new tasks or is pressed for time. These patients learn to avoid situations which require the processing of new or complex information. They tend to think in concrete terms. If asked to interpret the proverb, "A rolling stone gathers no moss," the patient is apt to say, "Moss cannot grow if the stone keeps moving around." That is an example of concrete as versus abstract thinking.

Judgment and impulse control commonly are impaired. There may be neglect of personal hygiene and appearance, and a man who has been a very prudish individual may begin to use inappropriate curse words or obscene language. There will be a general disregard for the usual rules of social conduct and such things as shoplifting or complete disregard of the rights of others may occur. Judgment is particularly impaired when there is some disease process involving the frontal lobes of the brain.

Personality change almost invariably is present in Dementia and frequently consists of an accentuation of previous personality traits. A quiet sort of person is apt to become more apathetic and withdrawn, but irritability and quick changes of mood are characteristic. A person who has been very pleasant and agreeable may become extremely agitated and difficult. Many patients become oversuspicious and distrustful of those closest to them as they lose the ability to process incoming information correctly.

Primary Degenerative Dementia (Alzheimer's) is the most common Dementia. The condition also can be due to central nervous system infections of any kind, brain trauma, toxic-metabolic disturbances such as pernicious anemia, hypothyroidism, bromide intoxication, vascular disease, and neurological diseases such as Huntington's Chorea. The condition is most common in elderly people but, in its early phases, it may be difficult to differentiate from depression. This must be kept in mind since depression is a reversible condition.

Diagnostic Criteria for Dementia

A. Loss of intellectual abilities sufficient to interfere with social or occupational functioning.
B. Memory impairment.
C. At least one of the following:
    1. impairment of abstract thinking
    2. impaired judgment

3. other disturbances of higher cortical function such as language disorder (aphasia), inability to carry out motor activities (apraxia), or failure to recognize or identify objects despite intact sensory function (agnosia)
4. personality changes

D. State of consciousness not clouded so as to meet the criteria for delirium or intoxication.

E. Evidence from history, physical, or laboratory examinations of a specific organic disorder and/or some organic factor necessary for the development of the syndrome is presumed to be present.

Amnestic Syndrome

This refers to an impairment in short-and long-term memory occurring in an otherwise normal state of consciousness. These people have both an ongoing inability to learn new material and an inability to recall information previously known. Frequently, memories of the very remote past are recalled better than those that occurred yesterday. The patients may use imaginary events to fill in gaps in memory (confabulations), and most will demonstrate apathy, lack of initiative, and emotional blandness so that they appear unconcerned over their condition.

Amnestic Syndrome can be caused by any pathological process that produces bilateral damage to certain areas of the brain, primarily the limbic system. It can be caused by trauma, surgical operations, lack of oxygen for several minutes, strokes, and some infections. One of the most common forms of Amnestic Syndrome is associated with thiamine deficiency due to the chronic use of alcohol (Korsakoff Syndrome). This condition, somewhat more prevalent in women, is an important medical problem.

Case Example

J.M. was a 56-year-old pharmacist and civic leader in his community. Few people knew that he had been drinking over two pints of vodka daily for many years. His family had noted some changes in his personality, but were not alarmed until he urinated on the floor of his busy pharmacy one morning.

Mr. M. was hospitalized for a complete workup which revealed only the mental symptoms of inability to abstract, memory loss, poor judgment, and a complete unconcern for his condition. When asked about the incident of urination in the pharmacy, he denied it and stated that he had spent that morning in conference with the Governor (confabulation).

Diagnostic Criteria for Amnestic Syndrome

A. Short- and long-term memory impairment.
B. No clouding of consciousness or general loss of intellectual abilities.
C. Evidence from the examinations of a specific organic factor judged to be the cause of or related to the disturbance.

Organic Delusional Syndrome

This refers to the presence of delusions that occur in a normal state of consciousness and that are due to a specific organic factor. The delusions can be quite variable and depend to some extent on the cause. The most common types of false beliefs are those of persecution. Hallucinations may or may not be present. Many other symptoms such as rambling or incoherent speech and abnormalities of the emotions may be present, depending upon the severity of the condition.

Many conditions can cause Organic Delusional Syndrome, but one of the most common is drug abuse. Amphetamines are particularly liable to produce a syndrome that looks like acute Schizophrenia with delusions, but any one of the many hallucinogenic drugs may be the cause.

The condition is called Organic Hallucinosis when hallucinations are the dominant feature. The patient expresses true fear of the hallucinations: delusions, if present, will be related to the hallucinations.

Diagnostic Criteria for Organic Delusional Syndrome

A. Delusions are the predominant clinical feature.

B. There is no clouding of consciousness, no significant loss of intellectual abilities, and no prominent hallucinations.
C. There is evidence of a specific organic factor judged to be the cause.

Organic Hallucinosis

The necessary feature of this condition is the presence of persistent or recurrent hallucinations that occur in a normal state of consciousness and that are caused by a specific organic factor. The hallucinations may be auditory, visual, or involve taste, smell, or touch. Hallucinogenic drugs are most apt to produce visual hallucinations, but alcohol is more apt to produce auditory hallucinations or a mixture of both auditory and visual. The patient may be aware that the hallucinations are unreal or may be quite convinced of their reality and be very frightened.

Even though drugs and alcohol are the main causes, this condition also can be due to temporal lobe seizures and/or sensory deprivation. The symptoms are apt to be temporary in these conditions.

Diagnostic Criteria for Organic Hallucinosis

A. Persistent or recurrent hallucinations.
B. No clouding of consciousness; no significant loss of intellectual abilities; no predominant disturbance of mood; no predominant delusions.
C. Evidence of a specific organic factor judged to be the cause.

Organic Affective Syndrome

The essential feature is a disturbance of mood resembling either a manic episode or a depressive episode, but due to a specific organic factor. The degree of the disturbance may range from mild to severe and may look very much like true manic-depression (Bipolar Disorder). If the patient is depressed the symptoms may include fearfulness, anxiety, irritability, and excessive concern about body functions. There may be feelings of persecution and worthlessness. If the mood is manic the patient may be euphoric, irritable, and overactive.

Organic Affective Syndrome usually is caused by toxic or metabolic conditions. Many drugs such as reserpine, methyldopa, hallucinogens, and some viral infections of the brain may be the cause. Disorders of the thyroid, parathyroids, and the adrenal glands have been implicated.

Diagnostic Criteria for Organic Affective Syndrome

A. The main disturbance is in mood with at least two of the symptoms of manic or major depressive episode.
B. There is no clouding of consciousness; no predominant delusions or hallucinations.
C. There is evidence of a specific organic factor judged to be the cause.

Organic Personality Syndrome

This is a condition marked by a change in personality due to a specific organic factor, but not due to any of the above discussed brain syndromes. The clinical signs and symptoms depend primarily on the nature and the localization of the disease process in the brain. One most frequently sees an increased emotional lability (marked fluctuation) and impairment in impulse control and/or social judgment. There may be outbursts of temper and belligerancy, bouts of crying without provocation, socially inappropriate actions such as sexual indiscretions. Most of these episodes will not concern the patient appropriately. The patient may lose interest in previous hobbies and avocations and show little concern about the practical aspects of living.

This condition previously was called the "frontal lobe syndrome" when the damage specifically was in the frontal part of the cortex.

Occasionally, the Organic Personality Syndrome is one of the first signs of developing Dementia or a disease such as Multiple Sclerosis. The degree of impairment is variable and may or may not be progressive.

The etiology usually is a structural damage to the frontal lobe cortex. It can vary from a meningioma (benign brain tumor) pressing on the frontal lobes to accidental trauma or to blood vessel disease or malformation.

The differential diagnosis depends upon the predominant symptoms. There also will be significant loss of intellectual abilities and this may signal the early onset of Dementia. Affective changes will occur as in the Organic Affective Syndrome but, again, these will not be the dominant symptoms.

Case Example

A Korean War Veteran, a college graduate whose I.Q. had been 115, worked as a laundry helper in a V.A. hospital. His major symptoms were silly, naive remarks, uncontrollable laughing spells followed by anger, and an irresistible impulse to pat females on the buttocks. He was unable to learn new tasks if they required long periods of concentration, but functioned well under direct supervision. He had been hit in the forehead by a shell fragment which removed part of both frontal lobes of his brain.

Diagnostic Criteria for Organic Personality Syndrome

A. A marked change in behavior or personality involving at least one of the following:
    1. Emotional lability as in explosive temper outbursts, sudden crying.
    2. Impairment in impulse control with poor social judgment, sexual indiscretions, shoplifting, etc.
    3. Apathy and indifference
    4. Suspiciousness or paranoid ideas

B. No clouding of consciousness as in Delirium; no significant loss of intellectual abilities as in Dementia; no predominant disturbances of mood as in Organic Affective Syndrome; and none of the major symptoms of Organic Delusional Syndrome or Organic Hallucinosis.

C. Evidence from history, physical, or laboratory tests of a specific organic factor that may be the cause.

Generalities on Organic Brain Syndromes

There are many subdivisions of Organic Brain Syndromes, frequently based upon the specific etiology. For example, one can classify them as Caffeine Intoxication, Marijuana Delusional Disorder, Phencyclidine (PCP) Delirium, Alcoholic Hallucinosis, Cocaine Organic Disorder, or as due to any intoxicating substance.

In general, the symptoms do not differ remarkably enough for one to make a specific diagnosis without a complete history; this most frequently must come from outside sources due to the inability of the patient to be accurate at that moment.

TREATMENT OF ORGANIC MENTAL DISORDERS

The treatment involves two phases: specific and general.

Specific Treatment

Specific treatment requires a knowledge of the specific etiology. This means a thorough physical and laboratory examination of every patient and, above all, a detailed history from as many outside sources as possible. Elimination of the causative factor may be possible as in drug intoxications and chemical and metabolic disorders, but in many instances, such as Delirium caused by brain damage due to strokes, the treatment may not be specific. Obviously the treatment will be less specific when there is traumatic brain damage.

General Treatment

This includes protection of the patient and those around him. Certain generalities must be kept in mind:

1. The patient should be kept in a well-lighted, quiet, calm atmosphere.
2. Whatever measures necessary must be taken to prevent the patient from injuring self or others.

3. When possible, only one person should interact with the patient at one time and this should be in a very calm and reassuring manner.
4. The patient must be given constant assurance as to basic reality factors such as time, date, place, situation, and so forth. This may necessitate repeating over and over what appears to be obvious to others.
5. Delirious and very agitated patients may require medication. This must be done only under close supervision of the patient since one often cannot be certain as to previous drug ingestion. Blood pressure and vital signs must be monitored no matter which of the tranquilizing drugs are used. Several are available and there is no great evidence that one is superior to the other. Haloperidol (Haldol), thiothixene (Navane), chlordiazepoxide (Librium), and diazepam (Valium) all have been used successfully.
6. A complete examination of the patient with adequate use of laboratory should be started as soon as possible to determine, if feasible, the specific organic cause.
7. And above all, speak to the patient in very concrete, understandable, firm, and reassuring words. Remember that you are the patient's temporary Ego (tester of reality).

BIBLIOGRAPHY

Fauman, M.: Treatment of the agitated patient with an organic brain disorder. *JAMA, 240:*380-382, 1978.

Hendrie, H. (ed.): Brain syndromes. *Psychiatric Clin. North Am., 1:*1. Philadelphia, W.B. Saunders Co., 1978.

Lipowski, Z.: A new look at organic brain syndromes. *Am. J. Psychiatry, 137:*674-678, 1980.

Terry, R.: Dementia: a brief and selective review. *Arch. Neurology, 33:*1-4, 1976.

Wells, W.: Chronic brain disease: an overview. *Am. J. Psychiatry, 135:*1-12, 1978.

VI

Substance Use Disorders

This diagnostic class deals with behavioral changes associated with more or less regular use of substances that affect primarily the central nervous system. Cultures and societies differ greatly in their attitudes toward substance use, but we will be concerned with chemically-induced behavioral changes which almost all people would view as undesirable. We are speaking of behavioral changes which include impairment in social or occupational functioning; inability to control use of, or to stop taking, the substance; and/or the development of withdrawal symptoms when the substance is reduced or discontinued.

These disorders are to be distinguished from the corresponding portions of the Organic Mental Disorders in the previous chapter. The organic conditions usually follow prolonged use of one or more of these substances and/or the abrupt withdrawal. It is the rule that people suffering from Substance Use Disorder sooner or later will have an Organic Mental Disorder such as intoxication or withdrawal.

Substance abuse alone must be differentiated from substance dependence. Three criteria distinguish substance abuse from nonpathological substance use. This is not always an easy determination in a culture such as ours which uses a large number of relatively socially accepted drugs such as alcohol and sedatives. Abuse is assumed when:

A. There is a pattern of pathological use manifested by intoxication throughout the day, inability to stop or cut down the substance, repeated unsuccessful efforts to control the use of the substance and, the continuation of the substance despite the fact that it is causing difficulties in health and/or functioning.

B. There is impairment in social or occupational functioning caused by the pattern of substance use. Repeated difficulties within the family or other social relationships, legal difficulties and/or evidence of poor judgment all can be taken as evidence of abuse. Most often, one sees deterioration in functioning at work or in school and these individuals frequently have shown previous disorders of personality or other impairments in social functioning.

C. The duration must have been for at least one month. It would be unfair to diagnose a person as a substance abuser on one or two episodes of misuse of a specific drug. Evidence shows that the majority of youngsters by college age have experimented at least once with one of these substances.

Substance dependence represents a more severe form of substance abuse and requires physiological dependence, psychological dependence, and some development of tolerance (habituation). The clinching diagnostic sign is a withdrawl syndrome, usually a temporary Organic Brain Syndrome, upon discontinuance or upon reducing the amount of substance ingested. Almost all people with a substance dependency disorder will have gone through a period of substance abuse prior to developing the end stage. Tolerance or habituation means that the brain chemicals have adjusted to the drug so that more and more of it is necessary to produce the desired effect. Usually, there will be the development of cross-tolerance for many of the other drugs. For example, a patient who has become tolerant to a barbiturate may be equally tolerant to many of the other non-barbiturate sedating substances and the minor tranquilizers.

Withdrawal symptoms do not necessitate complete cessation of the drug. A man who has been drinking two pints of whiskey per day may decide to reduce to one pint per day. A full blown withdrawl syndrome can occur in an individual who is ingesting an unusual amount of alcohol but has reduced his accustomed blood level.

CLASSES OF SUBSTANCES

Five classes of substances generally are associated with abuse and dependence. They are:

1. Alcohol
2. Barbiturates and similarly acting sedatives or hypnotics
3. Opioids
4. Amphetamines and their relatives
5. Cannabis (marijuana) (although some authorities question this)

Three other classes of drugs have been associated with abuse, but physiological dependence has not been demonstrated even though it is suspected. They are:

1. Cocaine
2. Phencyclidine (PCP)
3. Other hallucinogens such as LSD and mescaline

Prolonged use or even one or two heavy dose episodes of these drugs can be dangerous mentally and physically.

It is unusual to see a patient who confines substance abuse to a single drug, even though most will have a preferred one. For example, those who abuse barbiturates are apt to abuse alcohol, particularly when the barbiturates are not available. Opiate abusers (addicts) will use almost any and every central nervous system depressing drug available when the heroin is not obtainable.

GENERALITIES ON SUBSTANCE USE DISORDERS

Diagnosis of a substance abuse or a substance dependence disorder always should make one think of a preexisting difficulty. Substance abuse seldom is seen in young people who come from intact homes in which there is harmony and good communication. One also should suspect depression and look for other personality disorders. It is necessary to think about which came first—the chicken or the egg. Personality disorders and social difficulties obviously will be present after the substance abuse is well fixed, but it is important to know whether or not there was a preexisting difficulty which simply has been made worse by the substance abuse.

There are three main dangers in a Substance Abuse Disorder:

1. Delay in social and emotional development. This is particularly true of the younger person who, through difficulties with the law and the schools, fails to keep pace with the peers. The purchase of the drugs may require illegal activites and they almost always require association with undesirable characters. This can lead to severe social and legal difficulties which are not directly due to the drug, but are just as disastrous.

2. Organic brain effects. Prolonged use of almost all these drugs produces brain damage although we are not always able to identify it specifically. The damage is, in all probability, neurochemical in nature although there may be specific cell damage from certain of the drugs such as phencyclidine and the overuse of alcohol.

3. Physical difficulties. A number of physical illnesses appear more frequently in substances abusers. Alcohol overuse for a period of time can produce actual death of certain cells in the central nervous system which produces permanent brain damage such as the Amnestic Syndrome. The intravenous use of any of the drugs exposes the person to viral hepatitis and other forms of infections. Malnutrition and neglect of personal hygiene is extremely common, especially in heroin abusers. A major danger is that these drugs are bought on the street and one is never certain of the content. Much of what is sold as cocaine in this country contains little if any of that substance, but is a conglomeration of many other hallucinogenic and sedating drugs. The intranasal (snorting) use of cocaine can produce erosion of the nasal septum.

Perhaps most importantly, the use of these drugs leads to a separation of the individual from society with a much higher incidence of depression, suicide, and early death from a variety of causes.

ALCOHOL DEPENDENCE

The essential diagnostic feature here is the use of alcohol for at least one month so that it causes impairment in social or occupational functioning. There are three general patterns of alcohol abuse. First, there is the regular daily intake of large amounts even though the individual may never appear to be intoxicated. Second, there is regular heavy drinking which is limited to weekends and/or holidays. Third, the "binge or episodic" type in which long periods of sobriety are interspersed with heavy drinking lasting for days, weeks, or months.

The cause of alcoholism is unknown except to say, in a facetious manner, that it is due to drinking alcoholic beverages. There are interesting recent findings which show, without question, that there is a genetic component to alcoholism. Studies of adopted children have been done in several countries and have been controlled so well that it is now evident that the child of a biological parent who is an alcoholic has four to five times the chance of becoming an alcoholic by adulthood as compared to the child of a nonalcoholic biological parent. This does not change even if the child has been adopted at birth and never has had contact with the alcoholic parent. Just what is inherited, and how the genetic component works to increase the risk, remains a mystery.

BARBITURATE AND/OR SIMILARLY ACTING SEDATIVES AND HYPNOTICS DEPENDENCE

The essential feature here is the use of one of these drugs for at least one month so that there is impairment in social or occupational functioning. You can see that this does not differ from the criteria for alcoholism. Dependence on one of these drugs requires evidence of withdrawal when the drug is decreased or discontinued. Many of these people have begun the use of one of these drugs through legal prescriptions for insomnia or for "tension." Since tolerance develops very rapidly, the dose usually has to be increased periodically to prevent withdrawal. This type of drug usually is not begun in adolescence and is more apt to be seen in middle class individuals between the ages of 30 and 60 and more females than males are involved. The acute withdrawal symptoms are extreme nervousness and irritability, total insomnia, and frequently severe convulsions resembling grand mal seizures.

OPIOID DEPENDENCE

There is the requirement of at least one month of pathological use with impairment in social or occupational functioning. These drugs are far more apt to produce rapid tolerance and more severe withdrawal symptoms. Most of these people begin by a period of "polydrug use" which involves almost any of the nonopioid materials. Approximately half of the people who engage in opioid use go on to develop dependence. Once this is established, the individual operates as a true addict and this becomes the main concern of life. Now the drug is not taken to produce a good feeling, but is necessary to prevent severe illness (wthdrawal).

The death rate of opioid dependent people (and we are referring mostly to heroin) is extremely high because of the physical complications of the disorder and the life-style which is necessary to support it.

Withdrawl from an opioid follows a rather typical pattern. There is the beginning of anxiety and tension from four to 12 hours after the last dose which gradually increases to extreme irritability and an almost uncontrollable craving for the drug. There is shakiness and, after 12 to 24 hours, increased sweating; in another several hours nausea and vomiting. Muscle cramps of a severe nature can occur, and throughout all of this the patient has an itching, runny nose and reddened and sometimes tearing eyes. Severely addicted people, if untreated, may die from dehydration induced by vomiting and diarrhea. This severe withdrawal syndrome is fairly rare due to the low concentration of heroin in the drug as sold on the street today.

The methadone maintenance clinics do not cure addiction. They transfer the addiction from heroin to a much safer drug which can be taken once daily quite cheaply and with almost no adverse complications. It effects, in essence, a social cure and prevents the patient from undergoing the tremendous dangers of heroin use and the legal complications connected with obtaining the heroin. Unfortunately, the cure rate is very low unless the individuals are maintained on methadone for a period of years.

Several studies show that discontinuing methadone in one year or less produces an 80% to 90% return to the addicting heroin.

COCAINE ABUSE

Cocaine does not fulfill the criteria for addiction because the withdrawal symptoms are temporary and non-physiological. The major difficulty is that the drug produces a great deal of acute symptomatology such as paranoid ideation, suspiciousness, and irrational behavior. It also is a very expensive habit and frequently necessitates the person entering illegal activities to obtain the drug. Overdoses are quite common especially when the cocaine is mixed with other substances, e.g., heroin, which act synergistically with it. Cocaine is the "in" drug and gaining rapidly in popularity, especially in the middle and upper socioeconomic classes.

AMPHETAMINE AND SIMILARLY ACTING SUBSTANCES

The usual criteria of use for one month with impairment exists here. These drugs very rapidly produce tolerance and necessitate larger and larger doses. They are stimulants to the sympathetic nervous system producing increased pulse rate, increased blood pressure, a feeling of unreal energy and abilities, and frequent bouts of violent conduct, perhaps more than any other single drug. In very high doses, these people are seen in emergency rooms with symptoms almost indistinguishable from those of an acute schizophrenic episode. The differentiation frequently can be made by observing the patient for 24 hours and noting the marked improvement which would not be expected with Schizophrenia. Withdrawal usually consists of prolonged sleep.

Phencyclidine (PCP) is a dangerous drug, and although the evidence is still coming in, it appears that it is capable of producing permanent brain damage in a relatively short period of time. Such people, mostly adolescents and young adults, can become extremely violent and frequently are brought to emergency rooms by police. They require immediate attention and restriction to prevent damage to self and others. The use of antipsychotic drugs may be helpful in controlling the patient temporarily, but a return to the use of the drug is almost certain to produce a recurrence of the uncontrollable behavior.

HALLUCINOGEN ABUSE

This includes some of the drugs previously discussed, but LSD has been the most popular of these drugs. They produce visual and auditory hallucinations, frequently of a very frightening nature, and these frightening episodes may recur days or even months after the last use of the drug (flashbacks). These drugs are particularly dangerous for individuals with unstable personalities, and it is felt that they may at times precipitate schizophrenic episodes in people who otherwise might not have had them. The immediate treatment can be the use of antipsychotic medication or the "talking down cure." This means keeping someone with the individual in a protected and lighted area who constantly and firmly reassures the patient that the frightening hallucinations and delusions are untrue. The drug usually will be eliminated within eight to twelve hours under this method.

CANNABIS ABUSE

Much controversy exists about the use of marijuana. It has been used longer than man has recorded history in almost every country of the world and it is socially acceptable in many parts of our society, especially college campuses. True addiction probably does not occur, but psychological dependence can develop.

The active ingredient of cannabis (Delta-9-tetrahydrocannabinol) has a long half-life (up to seven days) so that it is eliminated from the blood rather slowly. Daily use means that there will be a gradual buildup of the drug in the blood and the brain. In small doses it ordinarily produces a feeling of euphoria and well being and, all too frequently, the false feeling that one has extraordinary abilities and talents.

Whether or not permanent brain damage can occur with mild use is controversial, but it is no longer controversial that the long-term heavy use of cannabis produces what has been called the "amotivational syndrome." This means a condition in which the individual is perfectly happy with the status quo and is motivated, more or less, only to achieve a state of "high" on marijuana. This is usually characterized by declining grades in school, by loss of interest in extracurricular activites, and by socializing only with those who are also marijuana habituées. Tolerance to the drug develops, so that more and more is necessary to produce the desired feeling. A major danger is that the individual on marijuana is not aware of practical inhibitions and limitations and may do very foolish things. The drug gives a sense of self-confidence that is not realistic.

TREATMENT

It is unfortunate that the treatment for Substance Use Disorders in this country is not good. First, it is rare for one of these individuals to volunteer for treatment. They practice the mechanism of denial so well that they do not sense anything wrong with them, therefore why should they seek help? They almost always must be forced into a treatment situation by parents or some other authority figure or because the drug is not available. Even then, the results are not good, in that a large percentage return to the substance use soon after leaving the treatment program.

Alcoholics Anonymous probably is the most effective treatment for the alcoholic. The "cure" rate for any one term of treatment is about 20%. Alcoholism and all other Substance Use Disorders should be seen as chronic, recurrent conditions and treated accordingly. Lecturing, preaching, cajolling, and threatening probably produce more harm than good. It is frequently necessary for the individual to get into severe trouble before the denial mechanism can be broken through enough to allow proper treatment.

The patients on drugs which are addicting will require hospitalization and gradual withdrawal and detoxification. This may take from three to ten days for alcohol withdrawal and up to six weeks for withdrawal from large doses of barbiturates. The tranquilizing drugs, both major and minor, may be used to alleviate the discomfort but care must be taken to prevent switching the dependence from one drug to another.

A recent addition to withdrawal treatment is reducing the symptomatic time significantly in narcotics addiction. Clonidine, a drug used in treating hypertension, blocks the craving for the narcotic and markedly reduces the withdrawal symptoms. It cannot be used for long-term treatment, but recidivism can be treated in the Methadone Maintenance Clinics.

BIBLIOGRAPHY

Blaine, J., and Demetrios, J. (Eds.): Psychodynamics of drug dependence. *NIDA Research Monograph 12,* USDHEW, Washington, DC, 1977.

Cohen, S.: *The Substance Abuse Problems.* New York, The Hawarth Press, 1981.

Council on Scientific Affairs of the American Medical Association: Marijuana, its potential hazards and therapeutic potentials. *JAMA, 246:*1823-1827, 1981.

Gold, M., Pottash, A., Sweeney, D., and Kieher, H.: Opiate withdrawal using clonidine. *JAMA, 243:*343-346, 1980.

Goodwin, D.: Hereditary factors in alcoholism. *Hospital Practice,* 121-129, 1978.

Mathis, J.: Psychosocial aspects of drug abuse by modern youth. *Medical College of Virginia Quarterly, 6:*187-190, 1970.

Progress and Problems in Treating Alcohol Abusers, A Report to Congress, National Institute on Alcohol Abuse and Acoholism. *DHEW (HRD 76-163),* 1977.

Vaillant, G., and Milofsky, E.: Natural history of male alcoholism. *Arch. Gen. Psychiatry, 39:*127-133, 1982.

VII

Schizophrenic Disorders

The world "disorders" is pluralized deliberately because it is possible that the disease we call Schizophrenia represents several separate, but related, disorders of mental functioning. They all have certain aspects in common, but there are marked individual differences in symptomatology, course, and prognosis. It may be that we are dealing with a continuum of severity or that we are seeing different chemical lesions manifesting themselves according to individualized personality characteristics. The common characteristics of the schizophrenias always involve multiple psychological and cognitive processes. There are invariably disturbances in several of the following areas: content and form of thought, perception, affect (mood), sense of self, motivation, and relationship to the external world. It has been said that a schizophrenic man changes the external world to suit himself and his feelings, whereas a neurotic one changes the self and the feelings to suit the external world.

THE GENERALITIES OF THE DISORDER

Content of Thought

The major disturbance in thought involves delusions which may be multiple and bizarre. The most frequently seen delusions are those which involve persecution and suspiciousness. The delusions usually refer directly to the person in a negative or derogatory manner and involve frightening and/or threatening content. Often there is the feeling that the thoughts are out of control and that they are being broadcast from the person's head to the external world so that other people are aware of them. Others feel that thoughts are being inserted into their minds or that thoughts have been drawn from their heads or that all feelings and impulses are imposed from external sources. In recent times, these delusions frequently have involved electronic devices such as monitoring of thoughts by television and/or objects in outer space. In everyday language, we would say that the thinking is "crazy."

Form of Thought

The most common example is called "loosening of associations" which means that ideas shift from one subject to another without any rhyme or reason and without the speaker showing any awareness that the topics are unconnected. In mild cases, the listener may have trouble following the person's chain of thoughts, but in more severe examples the thinking shifts without warning from one frame of reference to another. This can vary from slight loosening of associations so that it is difficult to follow the person's conversation to complete and utter incoherence so that everything said is incomprehensible. The schizophrenic speaker does not convey logical information efficiently to the listener.

Perception

These disorders usually involve some forms of hallucinations, most frequently auditory. They typically take the form of voices which make derogatory or insulting statements and which come from without the speaker's head. One should suspect that no true hallucination exists when, if asked about the location of the voices, the person replies that they are coming from within the head. Sometimes these hallucinations give commands that must be obeyed, but most frequently they are insulting and, especially in males, may be of a homosexual nature.

Tactile hallucinations (skin sensations) may be present involving almost any imaginable sensation, and somatic hallucinations may give the feeling that snakes or other undesirable objects are somewhere in the body. Visual, olfactory, and other forms of hallucinations may occur, but they are uncommon and should make one think of an Organic Brain Disorder rather than Schizophrenia.

Affect

The word most commonly used to describe the affect is "inappropriate." The patient may speak of a horrifying or sad situation with a look of calmness or even pleasure. On the other hand, something that should produce an affect of elation or laughter may produce a look of sadness or no change in expression at all. The voice usually is monotonous and the face frequently remains immobile regardless of the content of the conversation. This is very disturbing to others since we are accustomed to being able to look at a person's face and gain some idea of how that person is feeling.

Sense of Self

In analytical terms, this is referred to as a loss of Ego boundaries and frequently is manifested by the individual being perplexed about his or her true identity, the meaning of existence, or by some specific delusions as described above. The individual feels unable to control the environment and feels that the thing we usually refer to as self is beyond control.

Volition

The lack of volition means that these people invariably show a deterioration in work, school, and social activities. Very few objects or events are of interest to the patient and goal-directed activities become virtually impossible. This lack of motivation may persist after the acute symptoms have cleared and is a hallmark of chronic Schizophrenia.

Relationship to the External World

The schizophrenic individual is preoccupied with egocentric and illogical ideas and fantasies at the expense of involvement with the external world. In the most severe aspect, this is called Autism, which means that the individual has lost the normal ability to differentiate fact from fantasy. All things are related directly to the person and all things have private meanings which make no sense to friends and relatives.

Psychomotor Behavior

This can vary from marked euphoria and hyperactivity even to the level of violence to complete and utter withdrawal. Ordinarily, one sees a reduction in spontaneous movements and activity. The most extreme type of this is known as Catatonia, a situation in which the person may assume a rigid posture and resist all efforts to be moved from it. These people usually are mute and unresponsive to all forms of communication.

Associated Features

Almost anything can occur in Schizophrenia, including pacing back and forth for hour upon hour, extreme immobility for indefinite periods of time, rituals of all sorts which make little or no sense, feelings of having parts of the body missing, and so forth. In most instances, there is no evidence of great disorientation in in Schizophrenia, but in extreme forms the patient may be totally confused and have marked memory impairment.

Schizophrenia typically begins during adolescence or early adulthood. Signs of Schizophrenia first noted in an otherwise relatively normal person after the age of 35 should make one think seriously of some form of Organic Brain Disorder.

COURSE OF ILLNESS

Schizophrenic Disorder cannot be diagnosed until the signs of the illness have existed for at least six months. These six months include the prodromal period during which the behavior may have deteriorated slowly even though there were no obvious signs of psychosis. The prodromal phase usually begins with a decline in the level of general functioning. Most frequently, one sees social withdrawal, a change in personal behavior, a loss of usual patterns of hygiene and grooming, a loss of a sense of humor, disturbances in communication, and occasional bizarre ideas or thoughts. Friends and relatives may note this change in personality, but frequently have difficulty in pinpointing the exact time of onset.

Once the patient has entered the active psychotic phase and has all the symptoms of delusions, hallucinations, and the other factors previously mentioned, the disease is obvious. There may or may not have been a known precipitating event, but most frequently it is difficult or impossible to specify a direct cause for the break with reality.

After proper treatment, there usually is a residual phase in which the acute symptoms gradually disappear, but the affect remains blunted or inappropriate and there is a considerable decrease in the ability to function as before the illness. There is a noted lack of motivation and these people are unable to focus the attention on tasks for any length of time. Full recovery from Schizophrenia can occur, but probably in only 30% or less of those afflicted. About another one-third will recover enough to continue reasonable function, but will have periods of overt Schizophrenia off and on throughout life. An unfortunate group of between 25% and 30% never recover enough to function as independent people and many require prolonged hospitalization.

The patients with the best prognosis are those in whom there has been a very good premorbid adjustment, there is an acute onset, there is a late onset, there is some obvious precipitating event, and there is no family history of Schizophrenia.

The most commonly seen premorbid personality of people who develop Schizophrenia is described as overly suspicious, introverted, withdrawn or somewhat eccentric. Usually, they have been very "good" children and have been well liked by friends and family because they were not involved in activites which caused difficulties. They had few friends and associates and most frequently were described as "loners." There are exceptions to this: some have been very active and even perhaps overaggressive people, but these are in the minority.

CAUSE

The actual cause of Schizophrenia is unknown. Twin studies and other genetic researches show a definite inherited component. The question is, "What is inherited?" In the general population, one sees a lifetime prevalence of Schizophrenia of about 0.9% to 1%. However, when one parent is schizophrenic the prevalence over the lifetime jumps to 9% to 14% for the children. If both parents are schizophrenic, this prevalence leaps to a high of 40% to 45%.

The evidence points to a disorder of dopamine metabolism in the brain. Do these individuals produce too much dopamine? Is it not broken down or metabolized rapidly enough? Is the dopamine of a different character? Are the thalamic nuclei hypersensitive to dopamine? These are unknown factors but, since dopamine is one of the major transmitters between the neurons in the brain, the connection appears fairly definite. The medications which have the most effect on schizophrenic symptoms are those which block the uptake of dopamine in certain areas of the limbic system of the brain, particularly in the thalamus.

Diagnostic Criteria for Schizophrenic Disorder

A. At least one of the following must be present during the phase of the illness:
   1. Bizarre delusions such as being controlled by external forces, thought broadcasting, thought insertion, or thought withdrawal
   2. Somatic, grandiose, religious or other delusions without persecutory or jealous content
   3. Delusions with persecutory or jealous content if accompanied by hallucinations of any type
   4. Auditory hallucinations
   5. Incoherence, marked loosening of associations, illogical thinking, or great poverty of thought content if associated with one of the following:
      a. Blunted, flat, or inappropriate affect
      b. Delusions or hallucinations
      c. Catatonic or other grossly disturbed behavior

B. Deterioration from a previous level of functioning.

C. Duration: Continuous signs of the illness and its prodromal phase for at least six months. The prodromal phase must have shown clear deterioration of functioning before the active phase of the illness began.

D. The depressive or manic syndromes (to be discussed later), if present at all, must develop after the psychotic symptoms or be brief in duration.

E. Onset before age 45.

F. Not due to any organic mental disorder.

Case Example

A classical example of the development of Schizophrenia is a 17-year-old high school boy who had never had a close friend in his life. He was a hardworking "loner" whose only activities outside the home were a paper route and school, where he made above average grades. He was involved in no extracurricular activities at school and his hobbies were listening to records, reading, and attending movies alone.

His good grades began to deteriorate noticeably in the middle of his third year in high school. He began writing inappropriate notes to a girl in his class in which he expressed his extreme devotion to her and told her that he was willing to change his religion to Catholicism because he knew that she could not marry him unless he did so. The girl ignored his letters, but he continued to write several each day.

The deterioration in his grades and the complaints of the girl to one of the teachers led to a conference with his parents. He admitted his great love for the girl and stated calmly and without emotion that he knew that she returned his love but was unable to express it because of the differences in their religions.

He was brought for psychiatric consultation and quickly stated that he was related to one of the leading baseball players (a delusion), and that he was slated to become one of the great stars in the baseball world. He could speak for five minutes without stopping, cover 10 to 15 different topics, and show little or no connection between any two of them. During this time, he might laugh or look sad, but his facial expression seldom matched the content of his speech. He denied any form of illness and said that most of the people around him were crazy, especially his parents, because they could not understand his logic. He felt that his mother was his chief enemy since he had almost certain evidence that she had not wanted him to be born. He would or could not produce the alleged evidence to support his belief.

The young man was hospitalized and placed on an antipsychotic drug. Over the next four weeks, he began to speak more and more logically and to question whether or not all his previous thoughts were real. He was discharged after four months of intensive treatment, but returned to school with no motivation to study and was soon unable to continue in regular courses. Two years later he remains unable to keep a job full time or to continue in school, although he shows none of the bizarre symptoms of the acute schizophrenic episode. He remains on a low dose of an antipsychotic drug and attempts to withdraw it have resulted in an acute exacerbation of his symptoms.

TYPES OF SCHIZOPHRENIA

Disorganized Type

This type, once called Hebephrenic, is characterized by marked incoherence and flat, totally incongruous or silly affect. The delusions are not systematized, frequently disorganized to the point of incoherence, and the hallucinations show no organized content or any consistent theme. There may be grimaces, mannerisms, all sorts of hypochondriacal complaints, and complete and utter social withdrawal. Every sort of oddity of behavior can be seen and these are people whom we think of as being totally "crazy."

When this type begins in adolescence after a history of being a loner, the prognosis is bad. It may be the end result of chornic Schizophrenia, and almost all these people require lifelong institutionalization.

Diagnostic Criteria for Disorganized Type

A. Frequent incoherence
B. Absense of systematized delusions
C. Blunted, inappropriate, and/or silly affect

Catatonic Type

The characteristic of this type is a psychomotor disturbance which may vary from total stupor to maniacal, aggressive excitement. There may be rapid alterations between the stupor and the excitement, or either condition may exist for several weeks. These people are subject to stereotypic mannerisms and something called "waxy flexibility." This means that if one attempts to move an arm or a leg it feels like bending a warm candle or a soft lead pipe. Usually, they are mute or if they speak, the content is incoherent.

This type was common in this country even two decades ago, but for some reason it has become relatively rare.

Diagnostic Criteria for Catatonic Type

A type of Schizophrenia dominated by any of the following:

1. Catatonic stupor (marked decrease in reaction to external stimuli) or mutism
2. Catatonic negativism (a complete resistance to all instructions or attempts to be moved)
3. Catatonic rigidity (maintenance of a rigid posture for unreasonable lengths of time)
4. Catatonic excitement (hyperactive motor activity of a purposeless and sometimes dangerous nature)
5. Catatonic posturing (the assumption of a bizarre posture such as standing on one foot with the hands spread upward)

Paranoid Type

This is the most frequently diagnosed type of Schizophrenia. The most prominent features are persecutory or grandiose delusions or hallucinations. One frequently sees extraordinarily inappropriate delusions of jealousy. These people tend to be unduly anxious, angry, argumentative, and sometimes violent. They may express great doubts about gender identity or fears of being thought of as homosexuals or being approached by homosexuals. This element is confined more to the male than to the female. Females are more apt to have the feelings that people are calling them prostitutes or accusng them of other forms of sexual indiscretions.

The condtion can vary from minimal delusional material and disorganization to severe Paranoia which necessitates hospitalization for the protection of the patient and others. It is unusual, but occasionally the delusional system may lead one of these people to be violent and even to kill. When this happens, it is the result of the delusional belief that the patient must act in self-defense or that a higher power has ordered it.

The onset of Paranoid Schizophrenia is somewhat later than the other subtypes, often not until mid-30s, and the features tend to remain more stable over time.

Diagnostic Criteria for Paranoid Type

1. Persecutory delusions
2. Grandiose delusions (frequently thinking of oneself as God, etc.)
3. Delusional jealousy
4. Hallucinations with persecutory or grandiose content

Undifferentiated Type

Occasionally, one sees prominent psychotic symptoms in a patient that cannot be classified in any of the above categories.

Diagnostic Criteria for Undifferentiated Type

A. A definite type of Schizophrenia in which there are prominent delusions, hallucinations, incoherence, or grossly disorganized behavior.
B. The symptoms and signs do not match the criteria for any of the previously listed types or meet the criteria for more than one of them.

These patients, when followed over a period of time, frequently develop the typical signs and symptoms of the Disorganized type, Catatonic type, or the Paranoid type. The undifferentiated period may represent an early phase of one of the more specific types.

Residual Type

The Residual type is diagnosed when there has been at least one episode of diagnosable Schizophrenia. The presenting symptoms show no prominent psychotic features, although there are definite signs that the illness still persists. One sees emotional blunting, social withdrawal, eccentric behavior, illogical thinking, and loosening of associations. Delusions, if present, are not prominent and may not be accompanied by strong feeling. Frequently this is called chronic or subchronic Schizophrenia.

Diagnostic Criteria for Residual Type

A. A history of at least one previous episode of Schizophrenia with prominent psychotic symptoms.
B. A clinical picture that shows no prominent psychotic symptoms as previously were present.
C. Evidence of the illness such as blunted or inappropriate affect, social withdrawal, eccentric behavior, illogical thinking, or looseness of associations.

TREATMENT

The treatment can be divided into the following sections:

1. Hospitalization
2. Medication
3. Psychotherapy
4. Rehabilitation and Resocialization

Hospitalization

Most people with acute Schizophrenia will require hospitalization in order to get the acute symptoms under medical control. The hospital environment will furnish needed structure and safety and, in itself, frequently produces an immediate reduction in symptoms.

Medication

Today's antipsychotic medications are extremely effective and one of them almost always will be given. There are many of these drugs and only a few will be noted here (see chapter on Treatment Modalities). The commonly used ones are chlorpromazine (Thorazine), thiothixene (Navane), haloperidol (Haldol), thioridazine (Mellaril) and several others. Each of these drugs appears equally effective when properly used, but will vary in their potential to sedate the patient and in their side effects. For example, Thorazine is much more sedating than Haldol even though both may be equally effective in controlling the psychotic symptoms.

The dose should be sufficient to control the acute symptoms, but should be kept as low as possible because of certain side effects. These drugs all block dopamine metabolism in the brain and, since they are not selective, they also block dopamine to motor control areas in the basal ganglia. This may lead to side effects which resemble Parkinson's disease. There will be a shuffling gait, flat facial expression, muscle stiffness, and a resting tremor. Drugs known as anti-parkinsonian agents (Cogentin, Artane, etc.) may be given temporarily to control these symptoms but usually can be stopped after 90 days. If at all possible, the medication should be reduced enough to eliminate these side effects, but that is not always feasible in acute Schizophrenia.

Most people feel that the medication should be continued for at least a year after hospitalization, but at the lowest possible level. There are some severe complications of continuing high doses of antipsychotic drugs over long periods of time. A condition called Tardive Dyskinesia may develop with involuntary muscle movements of the lips, tongue, face, neck, and sometimes of the entire body. This condition is more common in older women who have been on high doses of the drugs for a long period of time, but more and more is being seen in younger women and in males. The doctors frequently are faced with the development of this severe condition if the medicine is continued or with having the patient deteriorate into severe Schizophrenia if the medication is discontinued.

Psychotherapy

People with Schizophrenia have great difficulty in trusting others. It is extremely important that a close relationship be made with an individual who can follow the patient as long as possible. Compliance in taking medication depends greatly upon this relationship. The psychotherapy does not probe the unconscious nor does it analyze the early phases of existence. It is related to the here and now world and consists mainly in forming a trusting and advising relationship with the patient.

Rehabilitation and Resocialization

There are many forms of rehabilitation and resocialization, and some people will need to spend the days in an institution and the nights at home or vice versa. There will be group meetings in which the people learn to socialize with each other and learn to consider their illness as a part of their lives which must be tolerated. They frequently lack motivation, so very astute people are needed to guide them into some form of activity that is as productive as possible yet as devoid of stress as is necessary for a given patient. Decision-making is one of the most difficult things to ask of the schizophrenic patient and, until there is a fair degree of rehabilitation, this is to be avoided. In general, the diagnosis of Schizophrenia means at least a partial lifelong or recurrent disability with the need for more or less constant access to good psychiatric care. Total recovery with no residual effects is, unfortunately, the exception rather than the rule.

BIBLIOGRAPHY

Bellack, L., and Loel, L. (eds.): *The Schizophrenic Syndrome,* 2nd Ed. New York, Grune & Stratton, 1971.

Hansell, N., and Willis, G.: Outpatient treatment of schizophrenia. *Am. J. Psychiatry, 134:*1082-1086, 1977.

Heston, H.: Schizophrenia: genetic factors. *Hosp. Physician, 13:*43-49, 1977.

Lidz, T.: *The Origin and Treatment of Schizophrenia Disorders.* New York, Basic Books, 1972.

May, R., Tuma, A., and Dixon, W., *et al.*: Schizophrenia. *Arch. Gen. Psychiatry, 38:*776-784, 1981.

Silverstein, M., and Harrow, M.: Schneiderian first-rank symptoms in schizophrenia. *Arch. Gen. Psychiatry, 38:*288-293, 1981.

VIII

Paranoid Disorders

The word "paranoid" when used to refer to a person's behavior or attitude implies an above average degree of suspiciousness, wariness, oversensitivity, jealousy, hostility, and a characteristic tendency to accuse or blame other people for negative feelings or events. Paranoid symptoms are common in many psychiatric disorders from Organic Brain Syndromes to Schizophrenia, but this specific diagnostic group is reserved for those patients whose major mental illness is manifested primarily by delusions of persecution or grandeur and yet who show little or no impairment in daily functioning. This lack of major impairment in daily functioning is a necessary feature in the diagnosis.

The associated features shared by each of the different categories include a high level of resentment and anger which may lead to some form of violence with minimal provocation. Grandiosity, delusions, and ideas of reference are common and there usually is some degree of social isolation and eccentric behavior marked by an inability to trust others.

These people rarely seek treatment voluntarily since they feel perfectly justified in their feelings and attitudes. They usually are brought to medical attention by associates, employers, the law, or by relatives who become exasperated by the constant complaints and suspiciousness.

The conditions are relatively rare before middle or late adult life and they tend to become chronic with few if any major changes in the course and symptoms. Periods of stress, worry, illness—any upsetting event—may bring the paranoid symptoms to the surface.

The cause of these disorders basically is unknown. It is thought that they develop out of early life experiences in individuals predisposed to hypersensitivity and mistrust. A complete history often shows that there have been sufficient reasons for basic insecurity during those years when the child was developing a sense of trust in others and confidence in the environment. You will recall that this sense of turst is a very early developmental task, but that it is continuous throughout the dependent years. It may be that these people have suffered a series of rebuffs when they needed tenderness and love and that, over a period of time, they have transformed this need into a chronic feeling of threat and anger and suspiciousness whenever they truly experience a need for affection or closeness. This has been called "malevolent transformation."

Diagnostic Criteria for Paranoid Disorders

A. Persistent persecutory delusions or delusional jealousy.
B. Emotion and behavior appropriate to the content of the delusional system.
C. A duration of at least one week.
D. None of the symptoms of bizarre delusions, incoherence, or marked loosening which would lead to a diagnosis of Schizophrenia.
E. No prominent hallucinations.
F. No other illness such as manic-depression (Bipolar illness) or Organic Brain Disorder to account for the symptoms.

DIAGNOSTIC CATEGORIES

1. Paranoia
2. Shared Paranoid Disorder (Folie à deux)
3. Acute Paranoid Disorder (formerly a paranoid state)
4. Atypical Paranoid Disorder (You will note that this atypical category frequently is applied when there are the major symptoms of a certain illness, but in which there are significant variations.)

Paranoia

True Paranoia is characterized by a single well-organized delusional system that is permanent and unshakable in the face of all logic and which is accompanied by preservation of clear and orderly thinking in other areas of life. The person frequently thinks of himself or herself as endowed with unique and superior abilities which others do not appreciate. They do not consider themselves as sick, they rarely seek help without external pressure and then they do so with reluctance. The disorder is uncommon before the age of 30.

Case Example

A 48-year-old nurse was brought for psychiatric evaluation by the police. She had pestered them incessantly for over 12 years with requests that they help her prevent her husband from poisoning her, but she did not ask that they arrest him. She was convinced that her husband had been attempting to kill her by almost every known poison, yet she had continued to live with this man (who, incidentally, was a physician) and had continued to function as a very effective nurse in a large hospital. She maintained that her husband was a genius who had deceived his children and eluded detection by the police for all these years, but she also maintained that she was equally brilliant in that she had been able to prevent the fatal outcome. No amout of reason or logic presented over many years by the police, her husband, and three grown children had been able to shake her fixed belief.

Shared Paranoid Disorder

This diagnostic term is used when two persons—very rarely more—have a delusional system which they hold in common. The old term for this disorder was "Folie à deux," to indicate that it was a "craziness" which involved two people. It usually is seen in a very close relationship such as husband and wife or two spinster sisters who have lived together in relative isolation for many years. Ordinarily, one of the people is obviously paranoid with a delusional system of some type and the other is a very suggestible or histrionic individual who gradually comes to believe that the mate's delusions are real.

Case Example

A 60-year-old man believed that toxic gases were being surreptitiously introduced into his home by people who wished for him to move out of the neighborhood. (It was true that his neighbors found him objectionable, but only after he had begun to accuse them of wrongdoing!) He maintained that he could smell the gases very plainly and, despite the fact that a number of agencies had disproven his belief, he held onto it firmly. When seen in consultation at the insistence of the city officials whom he had nagged for years, his wife also agreed that she could detect the gas. She admitted that she had not been able to do this for the first couple of years of his complaint but, by the time of consultation, she shared the delusional system completely.

Acute Paranoid Disorder

The essential feature is a Paranoid Disorder that is of less than six months' duration. It is most commonly seen in individuals who have had some precipitating experience such as a drastic change in environment as occurs in immigrants, refugees, prisoners of war, or people who have left home for the first time. The onset is relatively sudden and the condition usually does not become chronic. The delusions tend to be unsystematized and there may be several of them that are loosely connected. The condition may be difficult to differentiate from a Schizophreniform Disorder (to be discussed later), but an important difference is that these individuals usually think and act fairly normally in all other areas of living and they do not demonstrate inappropriate affect. The course tends to be of relatively short duration, especially if the precipitating situation is alleviated and there are sufficient environmental supports.

Atypical Paranoid Disorder

This relatively rare condition is reserved for people whose main symptoms are paranoid, but who do not meet the criteria for the Paranoid Disorders discussed above. It may represent a form of depression, especially when seen in menopausal-aged females. If so, it disappears when the patient recovers from the depression.

TREATMENT

How do you treat someone who does not feel ill and does not want to be treated? Psychotherapy is the treatment of choice, but the difficulty is in getting the patient to cooperate. The therapist must be willing to tolerate a tremendous amount of suspiciousness, hostility, and resentment, but should keep in mind that the paranoid person is actually a lonely and very unhappy individual. It is necessary, at least in the beginning of the relationship, to maintain a distant and relatively reserved attitude and to let the patient decide when to initiate closeness and trust. This may take several months. The therapist does not argue or present logical evidence against the patient's delusional system and, above all, must never attempt to "trap" the individual into seeing the illogical aspect of the delusional thinking.

Occasionally, one is called upon to determine whether or not a paranoid individual is dangerous. This is a difficult problem, especially when the paranoid person has a delusion of being endangered in such a way as to feel that a defensive aggressive act is necessary. It becomes a matter of clinical judgment and, when there are overt threats of violence, the therapist probably has the responsibility to warn the proposed victim and to call for whatever legal action appears appropriate.

Antipsychotic medications may be helpful when the delusional symptoms exacerbate during periods of stress. A problem is that these people tend to distrust medications until they have a firm relationship with the physician. One peculiar aspect of paranoid people is that once they make a trusting relationship—a rare event—it is extremely intense and lasting.

The prognosis for these conditions, with the exception of acute Paranoid Disorder, is poor if one expects a complete recovery, but relatively good if one will be satisfied with a stabilization of the condition. Many paranoid patients can learn to keep their beliefs to themselves and to express them only to their therapists. They will not give up the delusion, but life can be easier for them and their families.

BIBLIOGRAPHY

Freud, S.: Some Neurotic Mechanisms in Jealousy, Paranoia, and Homosexuality. Standard Edition of *Complete Psychological Works of Sigmund Freud,* Vol. XVIII, pp. 259-296, London, Hogarth Press, 1955.

MacKinnon, R., and Michels, R.: The Paranoid Patient. In, *The Psychiatric Interview in Clinical Practice,* pp. 259-296, Philadelphia, W.B. Saunders Co., 1971.

Swanson, D., Bohnert, P., and Smith, J.: *The Paranoid.* Boston, Little & Brown, 1970.

Tucker, L., and Cornwell, T.: Mother-son folie à deux: a case of attempted patricide. *Am. J. Psychiatry, 134:*1146, 1977.

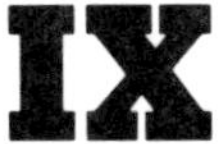

Psychotic Disorders Not Elsewhere Classified

These conditions are characterized by obvious psychotic symptoms, but they do not meet all the criteria for any of the diagnostic categories of the major psychoses. There are three specific categories:

1. Schizophreniform Disorder
2. Brief Reactive Psychosis
3. Schizoaffective Disorder

There also are some residual situations called Atypical Psychoses, a familiar designation by now, which do not meet the criteria for any specific Psychotic Disorder but which are serious and disabling illnesses.

SCHIZOPHRENIFORM DISORDER

A patient with Schizophreniform Disorder may show all the signs and symptoms of Schizophrenia except that the duration, including the prodromal period, is less than six months but more than two weeks. Some other differences from true Schizophrenia are the greater likelihood of severe emotional turmoil and confusion, a greater tendency to recover to normal levels of functioning and, in general, an absence of a history of Schizophrenia among family members. The condition may resemble an acute toxic psychosis or a hysterical episode carried to the extreme.

It is impossible to differentiate this condition from Schizophrenia without a clear history of the onset, duration, and the result of treatment. Many of these people, usually young adults, may be extremely disorganized and psychotic, but respond rapidly to the proper treatment and medication and return to full social functioning. This is not the rule for Schizophrenia, which tends to become chronic.

BRIEF REACTIVE PSYCHOSIS

This condition differs from Schizophreniform Disorder in that the duration of the disturbance is less than two weeks and that it almost always follows a severe psychosocial stressor—a condition not necessary for the onset of a Schizophreniform Disorder. If this condition exists beyond two weeks, the diagnosis must be changed to Schizophreniform Disorder or to Schizophrenia.

The symptoms can be as short as a few hours. These people usually are seen as emergencies in doctors' offices or hospitals and respond rapidly to the administration of an antipsychotic medication with or without a brief hospitalization. One should be wary of making this diagnosis unless some form of precipitating stress can be identified. The symptoms may vary from completely inarticulate gibberish and repetition of nonsensical phrases to suicidal or violent behavior. Delusions and hallucinations are common, but they usually are very brief in duration. The symptoms sometimes resemble those discussed under Toxic Psychoses and this diagnosis must be considered. It has been referred to in the past as "3-day Schizophrenia."

The condition usually is seen in adolescents and young adults. If it appears in middle or late life one should be suspicious of an organic brain disturbance, particularly one due to chemical intoxication.

Case Example

A 20-year-old female college student was brought to the emergency room at 11 p.m. by her house mates. She had begun to weep uncontrollaby at about 6 p.m. Within two hours, she was tearing off her clothing and destroying her room while screaming at "those lousy bastards" who apparently were torturing her. Her speech became more and more incoherent and she looked and acted terribly frightened. It took five people to get her to the hospital.

On the afternoon of her psychotic episode, this girl's fiancé of two years had told her that he was going to marry one of their mutual friends. Her first reaction had been calm acceptance and resignation. She had no family history of mental illness and no previous signs or symptoms of personal difficulties. She was hospitalized and given antipsychotic medication. All symptoms had cleared within ten days and she was back in school a week after leaving the hospital.

SCHIZOAFFECTIVE DISORDER

This is a much used and often misunderstood diagnostic category. It means that the clinician is unable to make a differential diagnosis with any degree of certainty from an Affective (mood) Disorder, Schizophreniform Disorder, or true Schizophrenia. The patient will show signs and symptoms of all these conditions at various times. One sees a patient who is either elated or depressed and in whom there is a preoccupation with delusions or hallucinations which are not congruent with the mood. These mood-incongruent delusions and hallucinations will continue to dominate the picture even after the main symptoms are no longer present. Many of these people, followed over time, will be proven to have Bipolar (manic-depressive disorder) conditions, but it is important to make a definite diagnosis as soon as possible. The significance of this lies in the effectiveness of lithium carbonate when one is dealing with Bipolar Disorder, especially in the manic or hypomanic phase, and the effectiveness of the antidepressant medications if one is dealing with a true depression. On the other hand, if the condition represents Schizophrenia, the proper treatment is an antipsychotic drug and a different type of psychotherapy. All too frequently this diagnosis means that the question remains in doubt.

ATYPICAL PSYCHOSES

The classical symptoms of a psychosis include delusions, hallucinations, incoherence, looseness of associations, illogical thinking, and/or behavior that is grossly disorganized or catatonic. The group called "Atypical Psychoses" demonstrates these symptoms but does not meet the exact criteria for any specific mental disorder. Examples are:

1. Psychoses with unusual features such as a single delusion of bodily change without accompanying impairment of functioning, a persistent auditory hallucination as the only disturbance, or transient psychotic episodes which occur only with the menstrual cycle. This category includes the competent housewife, mother, and businesswoman who becomes psychotically depressed for two or three days prior to each menstrual cycle. The psychotic symptoms completely disappear within a few hours after menstruation begins.
2. Postpartum Psychosis is a term restricted to women who develop psychotic symptoms which do not meet any of the ordinary criteria and which begin shortly after the birth of a baby. These women will show a mixture of symptoms that resemble an Organic Mental Disorder, Schizophrenic Disorder, Paranoid Disorder, and/or severe depression. The symptoms may begin immediately after childbirth or be delayed for several weeks.
3. There will be occasional psychotic individuals in whom there is not enough information for a proper diagnosis. These cases should have a deferred diagnosis and receive further workup and observation.

TREATMENT

The treatment of the Atypical Psychoses depends on the dominant symptomatology. Schizophreniform Disorder and Brief Reactive Psychoses tend to respond quickly to most of the antipsychotic drugs. The Schizoaffective Symptoms are changeable from mania to depression and treatment depends on the condition of the patient at a given time. The prognosis of Schizoaffective Disorder is not as good as that for the other Atypical Psychoses and recurrence is the general rule.

The symptoms of Postpartum Psychosis vary from abject depression to mania and the treatment varies accordingly. Recovery is the rule, but recurrence depends somewhat on future pregnancies. The rate of recurrence is high in women who have another baby in two years or less, but it is low in women who do not get pregnant again. The patient and her husband must be advised of the risks of further pregnancies.

Most of these patients will require brief hospitalization and all will need follow-up psychotherapy aimed to minimize the chances of recurrence. When the symptoms of Psychotic Depression are present, electroconvulsive treatment (E.C.T.) is very effective.

BIBLIOGRAPHY

Endo, M., Daiguji, M., Asano, Y., Yamashita, I., and Takahaski, S.: Periodic psychoses recurring in association with menstrual cycle. *J. Clin. Psychiatry, 39:*456, 1978.

Kasanin, J.: The acute schizoaffective psychoses. *Am. J. Psychiatry, 13:*97, 1933.

McCabe, M.: Reactive psychoses and schizophrenia with good prognosis. *Arch. Gen. Psychiatry, 33:*571, 1976.

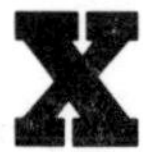

Affective (Mood) Disorders

This handbook follows the nationally accepted nomenclature of the Diagnostic and Statistical Manual III of the American Psychiatric Association. If that were not so, I would prefer to call these mood disorders, because it is possible for the affect, or outward expression of mood, of a patient to change several times during the course of a day even when the underlying mood remains unchanged. For example, a person in a very depressed mood may show anger, grief, or some other form of strong emotion.

To make the diagnosis of an Affective Disorder, there must be an abnormal mood that persists for at least two weeks. The mood of the patient should be in keeping with the expressed ideas so that a very depressed person will speak of losses, lack of pleasure, negative expectations, guilt, and hopelessness, while a patient in a hypomanic or manic state (elevated mood) will speak with grandiosity and sometimes with an almost infectious hilarity. Everything is bright and glorious despite the fact that the reality factors may be quite the opposite.

CLASSIFICATION OF AFFECTIVE DISORDERS

1. Bipolar Affective Disorder
    a. Mixed
    b. Manic
    c. Depressed
2. Major Depression
    a. Single episode
    b. Recurrent

3. Other Specific Affective Disorders
    a. Cyclothymic Disorder
    b. Dysthymic Disorder (Depressive Neurosis)
4. Atypical Affective Disorders
    a. Atypical Bipolar Disorder
    b. Atypical Depression

Bipolar Affective Disorder

This is the new designation for manic-depressive illness. It is characterized by alternating episodes of depression and elation. The diagnosis is reserved for patients who have had at least one manic or hypomanic episode. This requires a very careful history of past behavior if the patient first is seen in a depressed phase.

Cause

Hereditary factors are thought to be more important in this condition than in any other psychiatric disorder. Family studies, adoption studies, and long-range longitudinal studies of people show that there also may be a connection between Alcoholism and Antisocial Personality and Bipolar Affective Disorder. All facts point to the genetic component, but the exact method of transmission and exactly what is transmitted from generation to generation is not known.

Most of these people have experienced greater than average mood swings in early life. There may have been weeks or months of exceptionally good spirits and high energy followed by a similar length of time of mild depression or reduced energy. They tend to be extroverted, outgoing, sociable, and hardworking people. They appear to be motivated to higher than normal activity and production in order to win the approval of others. Many think that their outgoing and vivacious personalities represent overcompensation for unrecognized feelings of inadequacy and low self-esteem.

One sees an upwardly mobile family background in the typical case. Bipolar Disorder is more common in the middle and upper socioeconomic classes, but especially in those families which have risen from a lower socioeconomic status by dint of hard work and perseverence. The families have tended to be very status conscious and to give approval based upon the production of the child. Social concern and what others think about them have been more important than the emotional aspects of the family life.

There now is little question but that the Affective Disorders involve the neurotransmitters in the brain. Perhaps this is the part that is genetically transmitted. The major hypotheses concerning the disorders of these neurotransmitters are:

1. The catecholamine hypothesis in which these neurotransmitters are decreased in depression and increased in mania.
2. The indoleamine hypothesis which means that the indoleamines are decreased in depression.
3. A combined hypothesis which means that there is an indoleamine deficiency in both depression and mania with a decrease in catecholamines in depression and an increase in mania.
4. Another theory says that there are two kinds of depression: one in which there is a functional decrease in norepinephrine and the other in which there is a functional decrease in serotonin.

These chemical terms refer to the major substances which transmit impulses from one neuron to another in the brain. Apparently, they are quite specialized and they appear in concentrations much higher in one part of the brain than the other. For example, their concentrations, and therefore their activities, are greater in those areas of the brain which have to do with mood and feeling. Other neurotransmitters may be involved, but less is known about them.

Course of Illness

The first attack of Bipolar Disorder usually occurs before the age of 30 and may be either a depression or a hypomanic episode. The condition rarely becomes chronic and dissipates itself in weeks or months, but the patient may get into considerable trouble during this time. As many as 20% of the people have only one attack, but it should always be looked upon as a possible recurrent condition. The recurrences may be separated by weeks or even many years. The frequency of the attacks tends to increase with age, but the patients may live relatively normal lives between episodes.

The depressive aspect of Bipolar Affective Disorder usually is accompanied by psychomotor retardation. This means that the patient's facial expression appears extremely sad, movements are slow, speech is unproductive or even absent, and the patient speaks of severe guilt, worthlessness, and hopelessness. There may be delusions which are in keeping with the tone of the depression, as seen in an affluent banker who constantly and monotonously expressed the delusion that he was solely responsible for the economic recession in this country.

Suicide is an ever present danger. Often, the risk is greatest either at the onset of the illness or just as there is apparent recovery from the depressive episode. It has been shown that over a lifetime between 15% and 20% of people diagnosed as Bipolar Affective Disorder will end their lives by suicide. This is far above the expected incidence.

Hypomania refers to a form of elation in which the patient is restless, overactive, hyperenergetic, flits from one task to another without apparent tiring, and may be a general nuisance to the family and fellow workers. The typical findings are:

1. Flight of ideas: the patient may jump from one idea to another so rapidly that the listener cannot follow. The ideas will be changeable according to external stimuli. A sound in the street may make the patient suddenly speak of an automobile, but an opening door may change the focus rapidly to another topic.
2. Pressure of speech: Rapid, forceful speaking as if pressured to get out the words.
3. Psychomotor lability: the elated mood can change quickly to anger if the patient is frustrated or there may be fleeting moments of depression.

The hypomanic person is euphoric and the feeling tends to be contageous to those around, but brief periods of depressed mood can be noted by observers. There may be wild illusions and hallucinations, almost always of a grandiose nature. The patient may get into considerable personal difficulty during these grandiose episodes because of the impairment of judgment toward the overoptimistic, overconfident side.

Case Example

A 50-year-old very successful physician in one 48-hour period destroyed himself and his family financially. He bought $100,000 worth of worthless paintings, purchased a $75,000 boat and two Mercedes automobiles, bought over $25,000 worth of expensive whiskey for his colleagues at a medical meeting—all of this done before the family could get him under control.

The physician was brought to the hospital by the family much against his will. He refused to accept medication and accused all the physicians of being idiots who were jealous of his superiority and of the fact that he had overnight become a multimillionaire and was about to take control of the stock market.

This man had first been depressed when a sophomore in medical school 26 years previously. His personality had been Cyclothymic (up and down swings of mood), but at no time had he been unable to function as a very competent internist. It is relatively unusual that he had gone for this long period of time between the depression and the manic psychosis.

He was hospitalized and given injections of haloperidol (Haldol) 10 mgm every 30 minutes until his hyperactivity abated. He had a thorough check of thyroid, renal, and cardiac function and was placed on lithium carbonate and the Haldol was continued orally. He was considerably improved within one week and was able to leave the hospital at the end of the third week virtually in his premorbid condition.

Diagnosis

It may be difficult to differentiate hypomanic or manic episodes of Affective Disorder from an acute episode of Schizophrenic Disorder. It may take a careful history and some period of observation of the patient before being definite. This also may be true in the very depressed phases in which the symptoms resemble those seen in Catatonic Schizophrenia.

Case Example

> One young man was treated for Catatonic Schizophrenia for three weeks, during which he remained totally immobile and mute and showed every sign and symptom of catatonia. He improved slowly and was able to leave the hospital in eight weeks and to return to school, even though not at his previous level of activity. Three months later he was readmitted to the hospital in an extremely euphoric, hyperenergetic, grandiose state in which mania was now obvious. The treatment was changed from the antipsychotic drug used for Schizophrenia to lithium carbonate and his mood returned to normal within three weeks. He returned to school, functioning at his pre-sickness level.

This represented a case in which the original diagnosis of Schizophrenia was wrong and in which only time revealed the error. It might have been that a more extensive family history would have been helpful, because after the mistake was discovered the family admitted something they had not told previously: two close relatives, including his father, had been treated for Bipolar Disorder in the past.

Treatment

General

The immediate treatment depends upon the condition of the patient when first seen. The first consideration is an evaluation of the suicidal potential. Generally speaking, the greater the degree of depression, the greater the suicide risk. When there are extreme feelings of hopelessness and helplessness and, when there is little external support, the suicide risk increases.

The more the agitation, the more the suicide risk. Unfortunately, many of these people commit suicide just as they seem to be getting better and when physicians and families are relaxing. Suicide is rare during the depths of the depression, almost as if the patient did not have the energy to commit the act.

A family history of suicide is very important. When a first degree relative has committed suicide, the index of suspicion rises remarkably. The more the patient has abused alcohol and/or sedatives, the greater is the risk of suicide. The more impulsive the patient has been in his actions, the more the suicide risk.

The second decision is whether or not to hospitalize, regardless of suicide potential. Obviously, when the suicide potential is thought to be great, hospitalization is essential. Inability to control impulses and proven loss of normal judgment also indicate hospitalization. Milder cases may respond to outpatient treatment if there is a responsible relative and if one is certain that there will be compliance in taking medications.

Manic or Hypomanic Phases

The manic and/or hypomanic phase will require the immediate use of an antipsychotic drug and, since the patient may not be cooperative, the initial doses usually are given parenterally. The most commonly used drugs are chlorpromazine (Thorazine), thiothixene (Navane), and haloperidol (Haldol). One of them is given in graded doses parenterally with careful attention to the patient's physical condition, especially blood pressure, until the hyperactivity abates, then it is given orally.

The patient is given a thorough physical checkup and, if there are no cardiac, thyroid, or renal contraindications, lithium carbonate is begun in doses of 300 mgm to 600 mgm three or four times daily until the patient's blood level reaches 0.8 to 1.5 milliequivalents per liter (meq/L). This may require a total dose of from 900 to 2400 milligrams per day depending upon the size of the patient and other unknown factors of metabolism.

Lithium carbonate is continued on an outpatient basis with frequent blood level checks for the first several weeks, then at intervals of two to three months. It is a relatively safe drug, but there should be yearly checks of thyroid, cardiac, and renal function as there have been reported cases of hypothyroidism and of reduced renal function. How long the patient should remain on the drug is controversial. If there have been many attacks it may become a lifelong affair, whereas a patient with only one attack or with two widely separated attacks might discontinue the drug after one year with the advice to return immediately upon noting a persistent mood change.

Depressive Episodes

The depressive episodes may or may not occur soon after the elation subsides. Very severe depression with marked withdrawal may necessitate electroconvulsive therapy (E.C.T.). There is much controversy about E.C.T., but the truth is that it is an extremely effective and safe treatment. There is no danger of brain damage and adverse complications are rare when it is properly given. Its effectiveness is particularly noted in the most severe depressions.

E.C.T. may not be chosen and one of the antidepressant medications can be used. These medicines can be given simultaneously with lithium carbonate. There are a number of these drugs available and several new ones presently are under development. Their action is aimed at increasing the available neurotransmitters in the brain. Certain drugs tend to act more specifically on norepinephrine and others on serotonin. Rather than to go into detail here, a list of these drugs will be included in a later chapter.

Psychotherapy is an essential part of the treatment. Bipolar patients tend to stop taking their medications when they begin to feel well. Many of them prefer the feeling of euphoria that preceded their depression, and as one man, an Episcopal priest, stated, "The feeling of being God is tremendous!" That may put it very well; the manic patient truly feels as if he were God and many seem to be willing to trade normal living for the temporary delusion of omnipotence.

Psychotherapy should attend to the everyday aspects of living and to helping the individual work out the many difficulties that have occurred during the acute phases of the illness. Perhaps the most important part of the psychotherapy is the establishment of a relationship which insures the patient's continuation of the medication.

Major Depression

This diagnosis has been called unipolar depressive illness, involutional melancholia, and psychotic depressive reaction. We will refer to it under the newer designation of Unipolar Depression. The diagnosis means that the patient has not had an episode of hypomania or mania, but that there has been only one pole, the depressive, of the condition. If there has ever been a manic attack, this diagnosis is not used.

Diagnostic Criteria for Major Depressive Episodes (Unipolar Depression)

A. There must be a dysphoric (unpleasant) mood or loss of interest or pleasure in usual activities with the lowered mood characterized by severe feelings of sadness, hopelessness, pessimism, irritability, and inability to concentrate. There may be momentary shifts from one mood to another, but the major direction will be down. The patient may express any feeling from anxiety to anger with the facial expression congruent with the expressed negative feelings.

B. There must be at least four of the following symptoms present nearly every day for two weeks:
    1. Poor appetite (anorexia) and/or significant weight loss
    2. Insomnia or hypersomnia (ordinarily the patient can go to sleep readily, but awakens at 2 or 3 o'clock in the morning unable to return to sleep)
    3. Psychomotor agitation or retardation, perhaps alternating
    4. Loss of interest in usual activities including hobbies, work, sex, and so forth
    5. Severe loss of energy and easy fatigability
    6. Feelings of worthlessness, self-reproach, or guilt, sometimes to the delusional level
    7. Inability to concentrate or think well
    8. Thoughts of death, suicide ideation, wishes to be dead, or a feeling that life is not worthwhile

C. These symptoms must not be due to any of the other diagnostic categories such as Schizophrenia or Organic Brain Syndrome. Depression can occur secondary to any other illnesses, but will not be the primary diagnosis in that instance.

The incidence of depression tends to increase with age. It is more common in women until after middle age, then the difference between the male and the female disappears.

Cause

There appears to be a strong genetic loading toward this illness but, as with Bipolar Disorder, we are not certain about what is transmitted. There seems little doubt but that there is a functional deficiency of one of the neurotransmitters, probably norepinephrine and/or serotonin in the brain. Some researchers feel that losses such as those due to death, divorce, and other separations in early childhood predispose an individual to future depression, but only if there is the genetic substrate already present. In any event, one of the primary aspects of treatment is to attempt to increase the available neurotransmitters in the depressed person's brain.

The past histories of the patients with Unipolar Depression are not specific, but one frequently sees very hardworking, semi-compulsive, outgoing, socially involved people. They have been people who wanted to be useful to society and their families and who appear to maintain their self-esteem primarily upon what others thought of them. The internal level of self-esteem appears too sensitive to external stimuli. Eventually some loss or failure, even though it may be only a fantasied failure, occurs and the depression ensues.

Case Example

A female physician and academician attempted suicide in a severe depression at the age of 34. She had graduated from high school, college, and a leading medical school number one in her class. She had taken an internship and specialty training in a major medical center with the highest possible honors. She married a successful fellow physician and became a respected faculty member at a teaching institution. This woman was beautiful, intelligent, energetic, and had never failed to succeed in a single endeavor, yet she became so depressed that she felt life was worthless and that she had failed in everything.

How did she fail? She had failed because each of her tremendous accomplishments had been accompanied by the fantasy that people, especially her family, would love her more and would idolize her for her achievements. The fact is that each time she achieved at a high level they merely expected more of her. They took for granted that she was going to be number one in everything, and the expectations of euphoria and great feelings of self-esteem that she had had each time she achieved a success did not occur. She put it this way, "No matter how hard I work and how high I climb there is always another set of steps above me and I will never reach the top." That was the failure.

Treatment

As with any depression, the first question is the suicidal potential. This requires a great deal of clinical judgment and the suggestions given under the Bipolar Disorder section can be applied here. Added information can be obtained in the first interview as follows:

1. Ask the patient if suicidal thoughts have been present. The answer usually will be "yes."
2. Ask the patient if a method of suicide has been considered. If no method has been thought about and the suicidal ideations have been vague, one relaxes. However, if a specific method has been thought about and the patient says, "I'd use a gun," the next question is:
3. "Do you have a gun available?" If the answer is negative, again the index of suspicion can be slightly decreased, but if the answer is "yes," then the next question is:
4. "Have you checked the gun recently? Is there ammunition?" etc. If the answer here is "yes," hospitalization is mandatory at once.
5. Always ask about previous suicide attempts and/or suicides in the immediate family. No matter what the answers to the above questions have been, a positive answer to this question raises the index of suspicion. When all five of these questions are answered in the positive, the suicidal risk is great and immediate protective action is indicated.

There are three phases of treatment:

1. Hospitalization
2. Biological methods (drugs and/or electroconvulsive therapy)
3. Psychotherapy

Hospitalization is obvious. The patient should be put on suicidal precautions during the acute phase which usually means constant observation in an area which prevents the use of any potentially dangerous object.

Electroconvulsive therapy is indicated if the suicidal potential is thought to be great or if the patient is psychotic. Psychotic symptoms of delusions and/or hallucinations are indications that there will be a poor response to medication, but probably an excellent response to electroconvulsive therapy.

When E.C.T. is not indicated or not available, one of the antidepressant medications can be used in increasing doses until the blood level is sufficient. Blood levels can be checked in most major laboratories, but usually the symptoms and the signs of the patient will make this unnecessary. Most of the antidepressant medications require from two to three weeks to be fully effective and they never should be used for a lesser time unless unwanted side effects make it necessary to stop them. The specific drugs and their doses will be discussed later.

A form of psychotherapy called "cognitive" appears to be the most effective approach to the depressed patient. This refers to the tangible here and now factors in the patient's existence. One does not discuss the earlier emotional aspects of living, but gives corrective feedback to the patient's negative thoughts and feelings. It may be necessary to give the patient a rather stringent schedule of activities and to insist that it be followed to the letter. For example, every moment of the day may be written out on a piece of paper with actual times designating what the patient will and will not do at a given period. The reality factors must be pointed out continually when there are unrealistic negative delusions and/or hallucinations. It is better to have frequent, short sessions with these people than to have more infrequent long sessions since their ability to concentrate and pay attention is deficient.

Many of these people will require the antidepressant medication for months,and most psychiatrists will continue the drug for four to six months after the patient recovers. This has been shown to reduce relapses. There are some patients who will need maintenance levels of these drugs over a lifetime in order to keep the depression from recurring.

Other Specific Affective Disorders

Cyclothymic Disorder

This refers to a chronic mood disturbance of at least two years' duration involving several episodes of depression and hypomania, but in which none of these episodes have been severe enough to cause hospitalization or total dysfunction. The depressive and hypomanic moods may be separated by periods of weeks or months of apparent normality. Usually, these people will go through periods of time in which nothing appears to interest them and their usual activities and pastimes become boring. The up (hypomania) phases may be quite desirable to the patient because they have tremendous feelings of energy and can accomplish a great deal. The onset usually is early in adult life, and family members note that the individual has these periods of mood swings and come to accept them as a part of the personality. The condition may exist throughout life with no grave consequences, but it is a frequent precursor of Bipolar Disorder. When noted in an adolescent or young person it is good to keep in mind the risk of progression on to the more severe illness.

Diagnostic Criteria for Cyclothymic Disorder

A. Numerous periods, over at least two years, with some symptoms characteristic of both the depressive and manic syndrome, but none of sufficient severity and duration to fit one of the major categories.
B. The episodes of mood swing are separated by periods of normal feelings and activities.
C. The usual symptoms of depression as discussed under Unipolar Disorder, but to a lesser degree. The same is true of the hypomanic periods in which there will be an elevated, expansive or irritable mood, but the usual symptoms of hypomania are of a lesser degree and rarely lead to hospitalization or confinement.

Treatment

Most of these people do not require medication or hospitalization since the mood swings are not disabling. Psychotherapy is extremely beneficial in allowing the individual to understand, and even to predict, those things which will produce the mood swings and to learn to cope with them. Some authorities think that an antidepressant medication is indicated during the down spells, but this is controversial. The general opinion is to avoid medication if possible.

Dysthymic Disorder (Neurotic Depression)

There no longer is an official diagnosis of neurotic depression. The term "dysthymic" refers to a chronic disturbance of mood involving either mild depression or loss of interest or pleasure in all, or almost all, of the usual activites and pastimes, but with none of the symptoms severe enought to meet the full criteria for a major depressive episode. The diagnosis should not be made unless this type of mood has been present for at least two years and these are people characterized by friends and relatives as being persistently "down in the dumps" or "blue." The onset usually is in early adult life when these people become habitually unhappy individuals regardless of the reality factors in their lives. The course is chronic and the symptoms tend to make these people appear shy and/or unable to make positive relationships in school or at work. School performance and progress may be negatively affected. It is more common among females.

Diagnostic Criteria for Dysthymic Disorder

A. At least two years (or one year for children and adolescents) during which the individual is chronically bothered by symptoms characteristic of the depressive syndrome, but not of sufficient severity and duration to meet the criteria for true depression.
B. Manifestations of the depressive syndrome are relatively persistent or separated by only a few days to few weeks of "normalcy."
C. During the depressive periods a marked loss of interest or pleasure in almost all the usual activities and pastimes.

D. At least three of the following symptoms present:
1. Insomnia or hypersomnia
2. Low energy level or chornic tiredness
3. Feelings of inadequacy and self-depreciation
4. Decreased effectiveness or productivity
5. Decreased attention span and/or inability to concentrate
6. Some social withdrawal
7. Loss of interest in pleasurable activities
8. Irritability or excessive anger
9. Inability to respond with pleasure to praise and rewards
10. Usually less talkative and active than expected
11. An attitude of pessimism and boredom
12. Tearfulness or crying
13. Recurrent thoughts of suicide or death

All these factors should be with the absence of delusions, hallucinations, or other symptoms indicating psychotic functioning.

Atypical Affective Disorders

This category is reserved for those obvious cases of mood disorders which do not fit properly into any single category. There can be Atypical Bipolar Disorder in which there is a major depressive episode and some manic features, but not of sufficient duration or severity to meet the true criteria for mania.

Atypical depression is characterized by the symptoms of depression which do not last long enough to meet the full diagnostic criteria or which for some reason cannot be fitted into a single category. The condition can be diagnosed in persons who have had Schizophrenia from which they have fully or partially recovered.

Depression is one of the major causes for hospitalization in this country and some form of it affects at least 4% of the population at any time. It is the major cause for suicide and it may lead to many secondary conditions such as alcoholism, drug abuse, and/or life changes that are detrimental to the person. Of utmost importance is to consider depression in elderly people who appear to be developing senility. The incidence of depression definitely increases with age and the proper treatment of many elderly depressed persons has prevented hospitalization or institutionalization for what first appeared to be senile degeneration. It cannot be overemphasized that this condition—depression—must be considered in all eldery individuals regardless of the specific symptomatology of the case.

Depression is a treatable and usualiy curable condition. It is a true psychobiological condition in that it is caused by a combination of biological, social, and psychological factors. We are able to do a great deal about the biological factors and this has opened up a new field of research and treatment with great promise for the future.

Secondary Depression

A word about depressions which appear to be pathological but which, on the surface, also appear to be warranted. A person suffering a major loss may develop many signs and symptoms of clinical depression. It is important to differentiate depression from normal grief and mourning because the treatment is entirely different. Acute grief, a necessary condition following the death of a loved person, may last several weeks or months. It differs from depression in that:

1. The symptoms of grief come in waves while those of depression are more constant.
2. The grieving person can be temporarily distracted and feel and act normally for a few minutes.
3. The grieving person does not feel worthless and shameful.

Grief can blend into depression, especially in those with previous histories of depression or with genetic predispositions. This should be suspected when the grieving process appears inappropriate or too prolonged.

Depressive symptoms are seen frequently in patients with Schizophrenia, but the primary condition, Schizophrenia, should be treated. Antidepressant drugs usually are contraindicated.

Many medical conditions produce depressive symptoms. They include hypothyroidism, adrenal gland dysfunctions, some collagen diseases, cancer of the pancreas, Multiple Sclerosis, and a host of others. It is important to remember that each person with symptoms of depression must have a thorough history and physical and laboratory examinations.

BIBLIOGRAPHY

Akiskal, H. (ed.): Affective disorder: special clinical forms. *Psychiatric Clin. North Am., 2:*3. Philadelphia, W.B. Saunders Co., 1979.

Andreasen, N., and Winokur, G.: Secondary depression: familial, clinical and research perspectives. *Am. J. Psychiatry, 136:*62-66, 1979.

Beck, A.: *Depression.* Philadelphia, U. of Penna. Press, 1967.

Guze, S.: Early recognition of depression. *Hosp. Practice, 16:*87-96, 1981.

Johnson, G., and Leeman, M.: Analysis of familial factors in bipolar affective illness. *Arch. Gen. Psychiatry, 34:*1074-1083, 1977.

Kreuger, D.: The depressed patient. *J. Fam. Prac., 8:*363-370, 1979.

Nelson, J., and Charney, D.: The symptoms of major depressive illness. *Am. J. Psychiatry, 138:*1-13, 1981.

XI

Anxiety Disorders

Many of these conditions previously were classified as the neuroses. "Neurotic" remains a good term to differentiate these disorders from those in which there are psychotic symptoms, but the meaning is too indefinite and global for specific use.

Every human being has experienced anxiety. It is a very unpleasant feeling resembling fear both emotionally and physiologically. The major difference is that fear is a response to an external, identifiable threat, whereas the feeling called "anxiety" does not involve a threat which can be identified, or the reaction is highly disproportionate to the real situation. Fear warns of an external threat; anxiety warns of an internal threat. Anxiety, like fear, is accompanied by bodily disturbances which include:

1. Muscular tension
2. Restlessness
3. Tremor
4. Excessive perspiration
5. Pupillary dilatation
6. Rapid pulse
7. Easy fatigability
8. Some form of insomnia
9. Irritability
10. Difficulty in concentrating
11. Sometimes dysfunctions of various organ systems such as the respiratory or gastrointestinal

Free-floating, or pure anxiety, cannot be tolerated indefinitely and frequently results in the use of Ego Defense Mechanisms which are pathological, but which temporarily control the anxiety. The type of pathological defense mechanism used to control anxiety often identifies the specific diagnostic disorder. Anxiety can be displaced onto a specific object or situation so that the patient feels perfectly well except when in contact with that symbolic situation or object (phobia); then the symptoms of anxiety will erupt. In other cases, the anxiety can be converted into physical symptoms so that the patient feels calm and serene, but may be more or less disabled by the physical symptomatology (conversion). The person with amnesia has controlled inner anxiety by dissociating completely from reality and "forgetting."

The diagnosis of an Anxiety Disorder is not made if the anxiety is secondary to some other condition such as a mood derangement, Schizophrenia, or an Organic Brain Disorder.

DIAGNOSTIC CATEGORIES

Phobic Disorders

The outstanding characteristic is a persistent and irrational fear of a specific situation, activity, or object which produces an unavoidable desire to stay away from that dreaded object or situation (the phobic stimulus). The patient recognizes that the reaction is excessive and unreasonable and may feel shame and guilt, but is unable to control it. Many times the phobic (symbolic) object can be something that is rare or easily avoided so that the phobia is unimportant, but often it is something as common as riding in an automobile—a very inconvenient situation for most people in an urban culture. The Phobic Disorders are subdivided into three types:

1. Agoraphobia
2. Social Phobia
3. Simple Phobia

1. Agoraphobia

These people are more or less disabled by a fear of being alone or of being in public places from which escape might be difficult or help not available in case they suddenly became ill. This can vary from one woman who was unable to leave her house for 15 years to others who may, under forced circumstances, be able to carry on limited social activities. Ordinarly, these people become more and more anxious as they get farther and farther away from home. Actual panic attacks may occur so that the person becomes totally unable to function, and there may be temporary dissolution into a state resembling a psychotic episode. A crucial point in differentiating a phobia from a psychosis is that the phobic person always is aware of the irrational aspect of the condition.

Agoraphobia is one of the most common of the phobias severe enough to require treatment. Its particular disabling effect results from the person's inability to socialize and/or to work. When the situation is associated with true panic attacks it is called "Agoraphobia with Panic Attacks," but when the patient can carry on some reasonable activities without true panic, one merely leaves off the phrase, "with Panic Attacks."

Diagnostic Criteria for Agoraphobia

A. The patient has marked fear of, and thus avoids, being alone or in public places from which escape might be difficult or help not available.
B. There is increasing restriction of normal activities until the avoidance mechanisms dominate the patient's life.
C. The condition is not due to depression or any other known mental disorder.

2. Social Phobia

This differs from Agoraphobia in that the main symptom is a tremendous fear of being exposed to scrutiny. The individual fears that there will be actions which are embarrassing or humiliating and this leads to avoidance of contact with others. These people have difficulty eating in restaurants, going to theaters, entering public lavatories, and/or attending other social functions. There is an awareness of the irrationality of the feeling, but an inability to control it.

Diagnostic Criteria for Social Phobia

A. An irrational, chronic fear of a situation in which the individual is exposed to possible scrutiny by others and fears that there will be humiliating or embarrassing actions.
B. Significant distress because of the disturbance and the fact that the patient recognizes that this is an unreasonable fear.
C. Not due to any other mental disorder.

3. Simple Phobia

The characteristic here is the same irrational fear and compelling desire to avoid an object or a situation, but it usually is a specific object or thing rather than a situation or place. For example, one 52-year-old lady, very socially active, developed severe anxiety even by thinking about a kitten, and had decompensated into a panic state when put in contact with or in the same room with a kitten. Another person was unable to look at pictures of spiders and similar creatures without marked symptoms of anxiety and, when touched by a rubber spider someone had give her child, she became blubbering mass of fear.

It is not known why or how the specific phobia is developed in a given person, but it is known that the phobic object, situation, or activity has come to symbolize something very horrifying and frightening to the patient—probably some forbidden urge, wish, or fantasy from early life.

Diagnostic Criteria for Simple Phobia

A. An uncontrollable fear of, and an uncontrollable desire to avoid, an object or a situation (other than those situations discussed under Agoraphobia and Social Phobia). The phobic objects frequently are animals and/or high or closed spaces.
B. Significant recognized distress because of the irrationality of the fear.
C. Not due to any other conditions such as diagnosable Schizophrenia or Organic Brain Disorder

Anxiety States

Anxiety can occur at a time when there is no specific situation or object which can be designated as a cause. The symptoms are the same as those previously discussed, but there is no known stimulus present as in phobic situations. The patient may feel on the verge of death, experience great choking sensations accompanied by chest pain and a rapid heart and, if carried to the extreme, there may be actual loss of control. In a severe disorder, the patient may breathe so deeply and rapidly that carbon dioxide is blown off producing a blood deficiency of this chemical. This can lead to tingling of the hands, feet, lips, and even to unconsciousness and/or convulsions.

Panic Disorder

The most severe stage of the anxiety state described above is called a Panic Disorder. These people usually experience increased nervousness and tension between attacks, but can function very well. The condition often begins in late adolescence or early adulthood with no obvious cause. Some researchers feel that there is an inherited hypersensitivity of the sympathetic nervous system, and that being raised in a family filled with anxieties, tensions, and fears acts to make the hypersensitivity even more reactive. Thus, a vicious cycle is set in motion.

Diagnostic Criteria for Panic Disorder

A. At least three panic attacks within a three- or four-week period in circumstances that are not truly threatening in nature. The attacks are not precipitated by exposure to a specific stimulus.

B. Panic attacks are manifested by obvious periods of severe apprehension and fear with at least four of the following symptoms:
   1. Dyspnea (shortness of breath)
   2. Heart palpitations
   3. Chest discomfort
   4. Choking or smothering sensations

5. Dizziness, or unsteady feelings
6. Feelings of unreality
7. Parethesias (tingling in hands or feet or lips)
8. Hot and cold flashes
9. Sweating
10. Faintness
11. Trembling or shaking
12. The fear of dying or going crazy

C. These conditions must not be secondary to some previously diagnosed disorder.

Generalized Anxiety Disorder

This condition means the persistent anxiety has been present for at least a month's duration without any of the specific symptoms described above. Generally, there are the usual signs of anxiety, mainly those of autonomic nervous system hyperactivity. The patient does not feel greatly different from ones discussed under the phobias, but the chronic and relatively stable aspect of the anxiety is the key to making the diagnosis. Panic episodes are relatively rare in these patients and, if they occur, should lead to a reconsideration of the diagnosis.

Friends and relatives call these people "worrywarts" or "high strung."

Diagnostic Criteria for Generalized Anxiety Disorder

A. Persistent symptoms of anxiety manifested by symptoms from at least three of the following categories:
   1. Motor tension
   2. Autonomic nervous system hyperactivity
   3. Apprehensive expectation and extreme worry
   4. Hypervigilance, hyperattentiveness and constantly feeling "on edge" and irritable

B. The anxiety has been continuous for at least one month.

C. There should be no other mental condition and the patient should be at least 18 years of age.

Obsessive-Compulsive Disorder

This is a fascinating condition in which there are recurrent obsessions or compulsions. The obsessive aspect refers to recurrent persistent ideas, thoughts, images, or impulses that make the patient feel very uncomfortable (ego dystonic) but which cannot be controlled. The obsessions tend to be senseless and absolutely repugnant to the individual. The compulsion aspect usually comes later and involves rituals and activities that occur in a stereotyped fashion so that the obsessive thought and/or feeling disappears at least partially. The compulsive activity may make no sense at all, and it is called "compulsive" because the patient absolutely is compelled to perform it. The compulsive ritual may resemble a psychotic act, but the difference is that the patient will recognize it as abnormal and will express the desire to be rid of it. A psychotic person will support the act and deny that it is illogical.

The most common compulsions involve hand-washing, counting, checking, and touching. It has been recognized for centuries in literature, including the Bible, that hand-washing symbolically removes guilt. Psychodynamically, the element of guilt seems to play a major role in the development of the obsessive-compulsive personality. The guilt usually is not justified and may involve some innocuous and long-forgotten situation from early childhood.

Obsessive-compulsive people frequently use what is termed "magical thinking." They feel that thoughts are equivalent to actions, so that a child who has had perfectly normal thoughts of killing or harming a parent may later act as if these thoughts actually had been effective. Thinking is equivalent to acting.

The pre-morbid personality of the obsessive-compulsive individual usually has been one of semi-perfectionism, extreme integrity, stubbornness, frugality—in short, the type of individual who makes a very good worker, but not exactly an easy person to live with or for whom to work.

Case Example

A 24-year-old man, a firm believer in a very fundamental religion, was horrified one Sunday in church by the thought that the Virgin

Mary was a whore! This wholly unacceptable thought went through his mind over and over again, much to his shame and discomfort. He prayed, consulted his minister, did everything suggested, but the thought would not cease. After several weeks, he found himself counting the stoplights and keeping a mental record of the number of red and green ones between his house and place of work. The thoughts began to decrease, then stopped altogether.

He counted the lights each morning and evening, then after about two weeks, he arrived at work with a count of four green and five red lights. But suddenly he was not certain. Had it been four green and five red or the reverse? He became so anxious over the indecision that he was forced to return home and repeat the trip and make a recount.

Eventually, he was unable to make it to work as he became more and more unable to accept the tally of red and green lights until he had made dozens of trips. He had developed a full-blown Obsessive-Compulsive Disorder.

Diagnostic Criteria for Obsessive-Compulsive Disorder

A. Obsessions must be recurrent irresistible ideas, fantasies, images, or impulses which are alien to the patient's normal personality and which cannot be ignored or suppressed in spite of all efforts by the patient.
Compulsions are repeated, purposeful movements or acts that are performed in a stereotyped fashion, but they are not connected in a realistic way with whatever they are designed to prevent or produce. The behavior is aimed to prevent something horrible from happening, and even though the individual wishes to change or stop the behavior it is not possible to do so. Even when hand-washing done 100 times a day produces severe skin lesions, the patient will be unable to prevent the compulsive act.

B. The obessions and/or compulsions distress the individual and interfere with ordinary functioning.

C. The condition is not due to Schizophrenia or other major mental disorder.

Post-Traumatic Stress Disorder

This condition is characterized by reexperiencing the traumatic event, numbing of responsiveness to the external world, and a variety of symptoms such as nightmares, exaggerated startle response, inattentiveness, and some form of insomnia. This has been called "traumatic neuroses" in the past and was seen most frequently during and after the wars. Diagnosis requires that there be some extreme precipitating event prior to the onset of the symptoms. It should be an event that would produce significant symptoms of distress in most people; in civil life this includes rape, severe assaults, automobile accidents, floods, earthquakes, and other tragedies.

These people tend to avoid any situation that arouses recollections of the traumatic event, and the symptoms may become worse if there is some symbolic reminder of it. For example, a patient who suffered a Post-Traumatic Stress Disorder after being the only survivor of an airplane crash would become extremely upset years later if reading about a similar disaster.

There is some association with this syndrome and the "survivor's syndrome." These people tend to feel that there has been some special reason why they survived when others were killed in the original trauma. They may feel that a higher power has set them aside for some great deed or, in some instances, feel extremely guilty at not having shared the fate of their companions.

Symptoms may begin immediately after the trauma but it is not unusual for there to be a delay of months or even years. If the condition lasts more than six months it is considered chronic, but most of the symptoms will dissipate in less than that time.

Diagnostic Criteria for Post-Traumatic Stress Disorder

A. Existence of recognizable stressor that would evoke significant symptoms of distress in almost everyone.
B. Reliving the trauma as evidenced by at least one of the following:
   1. Recurrent and irresistible recollections of the event
   2. Recurring dreams of the event

   3. Suddenly acting or feeling as if the traumatic event were happening again because something reminds one of it

C. Numbing of responsiveness to or reduced involvement with the external world marked by at least one of the following:
   1. Markedly decreased interest in significant activities
   2. Feeling of detachment from others
   3. Constricted mood

D. At least two of the following symptoms that were not present before the trauma:
   1. Hypervigilance or exaggerated startle response
   2. Disturbed sleep
   3. Survival guilt
   4. Memory and concentration impairment
   5. Activities designed to avoid recollecting the event
   6. Symptomatology resurrected when exposed to things that symbolize or resemble the event

TREATMENT

Psychotherapy

Some form of psychotherapy is necessary in almost all Anxiety Disorders. This varies from intensive psychoanalysis in Generalized Anxiety Disorder to a more or less intense supporting relationship combined with behavioral modification in Phobic Disorders. The therapist must have tremendous empathy and be able to "feel" the intense misery of these people. It is necessary to have some understanding of the developmental factors and a detailed understanding of the patient's past history in order to make sense of the symptomatology.

Medication

There are no specific medications for these conditions but there are many drugs which help ameliorate the symptoms and produce temporary relief. In one condition, Phobia, there is evidence that some of the antidepressants may have a more specific benefit than previously thought.

Panic attacks may necessitate the use of an antianxiety drug (minor tranquilizers) for immediate relief. Smaller doses can be continued in severe cases, but it must be kept in mind that all of these drugs have the potential for producing tolerance and habituation with long-term use. Intermittent sedation may be necessary for those in whom insomnia is a major symptom, as in Post-traumatic Stress Disorder, but again care must be taken to prevent habituation. Antipsychotic drugs may be used in severe Obsessive-Compulsive Disorders when the symptoms are producing secondary dangers. For example, a woman who was washing her hands hundreds of times a day needed heavy doses of chlorpromazine (Thorazine) in order to prevent the loss of all the skin from her hands. The medicine did not cure the illness but it temporarily reduced the compulsion to wash her hands by about one-half.

There are many reports of good results in Agoraphobia with the combined use of psychotherapy and an antidepressant drug (imipramine or phenelzine). The relationship of the action of the drugs to these conditions is not well known, but their clinical effectiveness in reducing panic attacks appears to warrant their trials.

Behavioral Modification

This modality is most specific for the phobias. For example, the woman with the phobic reaction to kittens may be able to touch a kitten in only a few weeks by a gradual desensitization process. This can begin by having her imagine kittens, going on to seeing pictures of them, then to seeing the real thing, then to nearness, and finally to touching the animal. This is a simplified version of desensitization treatment, but it simultaneously requires a good therapeutic relationship with the patient. There are other modifications of behavioral therapy including biofeedback and aversion treatments, but these are more specialized and controversial techniques not in the scope of this book.

Other

Hypnotic techniques may be of benefit in Post-traumatic Disorders, especially when there has been a more or less complete repression of the memory of the original event. It may be recalled under hypnosis and relived in gradual stages. The hypnosis can be produced by the usual passive method or by the use of intravenous drugs such as sodium amytal or sodium pentothal. This is a treatment which requires great skill and knowledge of both the hypnotic technique and of the psychodynamics of the individual, but it may be extremely effective under favorable circumstances.

Hospitalization

Hospitalization probably should be restricted to the most severe cases. If it is possible to do so, these people should be kept in the mainstream of life and treated while functioning in their usual social context. This will be possible with most Phobic Disorders, but severe anxiety episodes and some of the severe obsessive-compulsive states may need temporary hospitalization. Obsessive-compulsive episodes have been known to last for years and to produce total disability; others may flare up quite rapidly or remain in a chronic state which makes living difficult, but not impossible.

Most people can recognize some or all of these symptoms in themselves to a minor degree at one time or another. An irrational fear of a harmless green snake is a mild form of a phobia. Religions frequently use compulsive rituals in order for people to feel "at home" and to relieve guilt. Many of us have experienced periods of apprehension and fearfulness, however briefly, for which we could give no reasonable explanation. It is a rare individual who will not have some minor post-traumatic stress following an automobile accident or any other life-threatening event. The question as to whether these conditions become "disorders" requiring treatment is a matter of judgment and will be related to those things discussed under the chapter on Stress.

BIBLIOGRAPHY

Agras, W., Chapen, H., and Oliveau, D.: The natural history of phobia. *Arch. Gen. Psychiatry, 26:*315-317, 1972.

Marks, I., and Lader, M.: Anxiety states (anxiety neurosis): a review. *N. Nerv. Ment. Dis., 156:*3, 1973.

May, R.: *The Meaning of Anxiety.* New York, Ronald Press, 1950.

Miner, G.: The evidence for genetic components in the neuroses. *Arch. Gen. Psychiatry, 29:*111-118, 1973.

Nemiah, J.: Psychoneurotic Disorders. In *The Harvard Guide to Modern Psychiatry.* A. Nicholi (ed.) pp. 173-197, Cambridge, The Belknap Press of Harvard U. Press, 1978.

Suess, J.: Short-term psychotherapy with the compulsive personality and the obsessive-compulsive neurotic. *Am. J. Psychiatry, 129:*270-275, 1972.

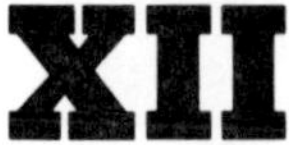

XII

Somatoform Disorders

This diagnostic group includes many conditions previously classified as neuroses or psychosomatic disorders. The outstanding characterization of them is that the main symptoms are physical (somatic), but that there are no organic findings or physiological mechanisms to account for the symptoms, and that there is positive evidence (or at least the strong presumption) that the symptoms are linked to psychological conflicts. The conditions differ from Factitious Disorders and Malingering in that the symptoms are not under voluntary control and the patient finds them very unpleasant.

DIAGNOSTIC CATEGORIES

1. Somatization Disorder
2. Conversion Disorder
3. Psychogenic Pain Disorder
4. Hypochondriasis
5. Atypical Somatoform Disorder

Somatization Disorder

The major characteristic is the repeated occurrence of multiple somatic complaints of at least several years' duration for which medical attention has been sought without any physical disorder being discovered. The condition usually begins in the late teens or early 20s and has a relatively chronic course. The patients present symptoms in very exaggerated and dramatic manners and frequently are seeing two or more physicians simultaneously and taking any number of medications, usually without prolonged relief. The complaints involve any and every organ system of the body and often begin in young women as symptoms concerning menstrual functions. It is a relatively rare diagnosis in males.

Many of these people should be considered for depression before the diagnosis of Somatization Disorder is made. The type of depression in which somatic symptoms are the main picture has been called "masked depression" and it is essential to rule out this diagnosis. A family history of parents and/or siblings with multiple somatic and emotional complaints is found often, and they have been called "medically oriented" families.

Diagnostic Criteria for Somatization Disorder

A. The history of physical symptoms of several years' duration beginning before age 30.
B. Complaints of at least 14 symptoms for women and 12 for men involving one or more of the systems listed below. To count a symptom as present, it must be reported by the patient as severe enough for medicine to be taken or for a physician to be consulted. The symptoms cannot be explained by any physical disorder or injury nor are they the side effects of other medications or drugs.
   1. Sickly: Patient believes that he or she has been a sick person most of his or her life.
   2. Conversion or pseudoneurological symptoms: This can include anything from deafness to semi-paralysis to convulsions.
   3. Gastrointestinal symptoms: Abdominal pain, nausea; a variety of gastrointestinal disorders are possible.
   4. Female reproductive symptoms: This can be anything from dysmenorrhea (painful menstruation) to excessive bleeding.
   5. Psychosexual symptoms: There usually is a sexual indifference at the very least and, at the most, pain during sexual performance.
   6. Pain: This usually involves back, joints, and extremities, but can occur in any and all parts of the body.

7. Cardiopulmonary symptoms: Shortness of breath, palpitations, and some forms of stabbing chest pain are the most common.

Conversion Disorder

This condition once was classified as a neurosis and was a very common diagnosis a few decades ago, but there has been a marked decline in the number of Conversion Disorders seen in recent years. The major characteristic is a loss of, or an alteration of, physical functioning that suggests a physical disorder, but which cannot be explained by any physiological mechanism. The disturbance is not under voluntary control. The classic condition suggests neurological diseases such as blindness, tunnel vision, anesthesias, parethesias, and paralyses. The symptoms generally involve the voluntary musculature and/or one of the major sensory modalities.

This is a fascinating condition to observe. One must think of both a primary and a secondary gain when evaluating these people. The primary gain is that the physiological symptom is able to keep some internal conflict or severe anxiety out of awareness. There usually is some temporal relationship between an environmental stimulus that is related to a severe psychological conflict or need and the onset of the symptoms.

Case Example

Two soldiers were returning from a patrol in Korea when they were hit by enemy fire a few feet away from their foxholes. One of them was injured slightly and made it to his foxhole, but the other was horribly mangled and could not make it to safety. The slightly injured soldier could not get to his friend because of the enemy fire and was forced to listen to his agonized cries for help for about an hour before he died. Sometime later when the fighting died down, the soldier surviving was found to be totally deaf. He had "converted" the internal conflict between reality (the danger of being killed) and the desire to help his friend into a somatic symptom: deafness. The symptoms of deafness was "chosen" to shut out the sounds of his dying comrade.

Secondary gain refers to the tangible benefits that the symptoms may produce for the patient once they have developed. The soldier was not able to return to combat because of his deafness and, therefore, was removed from danger. Simultaneously, he had saved his self-esteem and his desire to be a good soldier to some degree because the symptoms were beyond his control.

A striking diagnostic sign of a Conversion Disorder is called "la belle indifference." This is an attitude of calmness and indifference which is not congruent with the degree of physical impairment. Imagine a 17-year-old girl dressed for the high school prom who suddently develops total paralysis and anesthesia from the waist down. Such paralysis would produce extreme anxiety or even panic in most of us, but this young lady, suffering from a Conversion Reaction, was smiling and joking with the personnel as she was being examined in an emergency room. She was indifferent to her manifest condition.

The condition varies greatly in its severity, and many times minor conversion symptoms disappear without intervention. In other instances, the condition may last so long as to produce permanent damage due to muscle atrophy and contractions from disuse.

It is extremely important that these people have a thorough physical examination and all the necessary laboratory work. Certain conditions such as Multiple Sclerosis and other neurological disorders may easily resemble Conversion Reaction in the early stages. Once it is fairly certain that there are no physical conditions or physiological disturbances, it becomes equally important not to reexamine and to take measures which further fix the idea of a physical cause in the patient's mind. Most of these people are very suggestible, and they tend to be relatively unsophisticated as to anatomy and physiology. The diagnosis rarely is made in educated, sophisticated people.

Diagnostic Criteria for Conversion Disorder

A. The characteristic is a loss of, or change in, physical functioning suggesting a physical disorder primarily involving the voluntary musculature and/or sense organs.

B. Psychological factors must be judged to be involved in the cause of the symptoms as evidenced by at least one of the following:
   1. There is a time relationship between some stimulus that apparently produced a psychological conflict or need and the initiation of the symptom.
   2. The symptom enables the individual to avoid some activity that is undesirable.
   3. The symptom gets the patient support from the environment that otherwise might not be present, or gets the patient out of doing something undesirable (secondary gain).

C. There is assurance that the symptom is not under voluntary control.

D. The symptom, after a complete investigation, cannot be explained by a known physiological dysfunction.

E. The symptom is not limited to pain or to sexual dysfunction or due to any other form of illness.

Psychogenic Pain Disorder

The characteristics here are predominant complaint of pain, no adequate physical findings to account for the pain, and evidence of psychological factors that might be the cause. The pain frequently is inconsistent with the anatomical distribution of the nervous system or it acts similar to some known disease such as angina or arthritis. Most often one can find psychological factors that either cause or exacerbate the pain or which would make it reasonable for the patient to have pain in order to avoid some sort of undesirable activity or association. These people visit physicians more often than average and are prone to be taking several pain medications at one time. This last factor must always be carefully observed. They may undergo multiple surgical and diagnostic procedures, and almost always have visited three or more physicians attempting to find some relief. It differs from Conversion Disorder in that one does not see a lack of concern and calmness, and there rarely are total involvements of muscles and/or sensory nerves. It must be differentiated from Malingering and is obviously a great problem when there is some possible compensation involved, as is the case in minor automobile accidents which may produce muscle aches and pains which should dissipate within days or weeks. If there is the strong possibility of financial remuneration from an insurance company, these conditions may develop into a form of psychogenic pain without the patient being aware of any direct connection between money and the pain.

The pain also may be a punitive mechanism.

Case Example

A respected school teacher and family man had not had a single day for over two years without severe pain in the low back. He had visited more than 15 physicians and had undergone almost every known diagnostic procedure without a single positive physical finding. He was a man of high moral standards and a noted church leader in his community. He had become involved in an affair with a fellow teacher, something very foreign to his usual standards, which had produced tremendous feelings of guilt and shame in him. His psychogenic pain appeared to be a method of punishing himself for his "sin."

Diagnostic Criteria for Psychogenic Pain Disorder

A. Severe and prolonged pain
B. The pain is inconsistent with the distribution of the nervous system and, after careful consideration, no organic pathology or physiological mechanism can account for it. There may be some organic pathology present but, if so, the pain is grossly in excess of what should be expected.
C. Some psychological factors can be found which could account for the pain as evidenced by at least one of the following:
    1. Something happened which produced a psychological conflict or need shortly before the pain began.
    2. The pain enables the patient to avoid some activity that is undesirable and/or serves a psychological function such as self-punishment.
    3. The pain gets the patient sympathy and support from the environment.

Hypochondriasis

You will see that this condition may be difficult to differentiate from Somatization Disorder. It is equally important to consider the possibility of hypochondriasis being the symptom of another more severe disease such as depression or schizophrenia. However, when both these conditions can be ruled out, the essential features of this disturbance are unrealistic interpretations of physical signs or sensations as abnormal and a tremendous preoccupation with the fear or belief of having some serious disease. This unrealistic fear or belief does not give way to medical reassurance and causes impairment in social or occupational functioning. The patient is preoccupied with most bodily functions and may count the pulse many times daily, be aware of every little movement of the gut, be preoccupied with the smallest skin lesion or sore, and magnify every tiny sensation. They are typical "doctor shoppers" and both patient and physician tend to become frustrated and disgusted with each other. It is very difficult to keep a good relationship with these people because they soon develop a distrust of physicians and all medications.

Hypochondriasis is relatively common. These people have multiple hospitalizations and diagnostic workups, and they are typically anxious and depressed in everyday living. Friends and associates tend to avoid them since their primary topic of conversation is their bodily functions and dysfunctions. Some almost appear to "enjoy" ill health.

Diagnostic Criteria for Hypochondriasis

A. A characteristic unrealistic interpretation of physical signs or sensations as abnormal, with preoccupation with the fear or belief of having a serious illness.
B. Thorough examinations do not support a diagnosis which could account for the physical signs or sensations or for the patient's unrealistic interpretations of them.
C. The unrealistic fear of or belief in having a disease causes impairment in social or occupational functioning and resists rational thinking almost as if it were a delusion.

Atypical Somatoform Disorder

We reserve this category of "atypical" for cases in which the predominant disturbances cannot be explained by organic findings or for situations apparently due to psychological factors, but not fitting one of the above descriptions. This should not be a frequent diagnosis. These patients should be studied until they can be more definitively diagnosed.

TREATMENT

The treatment of Somatoform Disorders must be individualized. It is unfortunately true that the prognosis for this set of conditions is poor if one expects a complete cure. The exception to this is the Conversion Disorder in which the prognosis may be excellent if the condition is caught early and properly treated.

Psychotherapy

There is virtually no treatment for Somatization Disorder except good long-term psychotherapy. The major point is for the physician, usually a psychiatrist, to make a close personal relationship with the individual and to become an "alter ego." Most of them will be treated first by family physicians (usually several), but it is best if one person has charge of the medical care. It is extremely important to avoid multiple medications since they often produce secondary symptoms worse than the original ones. These individuals are susceptible to Substance Use Disorders which creep up on them as methods of controlling their discomfort. Their lives often are chaotic and complicated, and the physician again has the responsibility to give both guidance and concrete advice. It is necessary to be empathetic, but at the same time firm. These people do not "imagine" their discomfort; to them it is real. Analgesic medications must be given in minimal doses and watched carefully.

Psychotherapy with a Conversion Disorder is urgent in that the longer the conversion symptom exists, the more difficult it is to eliminate it. This is one of the conditions in which hypnosis may be of immediate benefit. Fortunately, most of these people are easily hypnotized, and the crippling dysfunction can be removed totally or partially. Many feel that the symptoms should not be removed 100% in order to keep the patient under observation and to get the patient into some form of treatment which will prevent a recurrence. For example, a total paralysis from the waist down may be removed easily by hypnosis, but it would be good to leave numbness or paralysis of a toe or a side of a foot, a symptom which would insure the patient's return.

The psychotherapy must involve closely the originating event (primary gain), but also must eliminate the secondary gain. Elimination of the secondary gain will require consultation and cooperation with the major family members, employers, and/or other associates. The more the family members and associates treat the individual as "sick and crippled," the more difficult it will be to remove the condition. Medications rarely are of benefit.

Psychogenic Pain Disorder requires the same type of psychotherapy as for Somatization Disorder, but will center more directly around the pain itself and those things which bring it on or exacerbate it. One looks particularly for reasons for self-punishment and for signs of secondary gain which must be dealt with as soon as possible. These people will have been to many physicians, and many will be referred to major medical centers which have clinics devoted strictly to pain problems. There a complete workup is given and some form of treatment program is outlined. It is good to discourage the patient from doctor shopping and going from one clinic to another, since this is not only expensive but delays definitive treatment.

These people must be protected from overuse of narcotic analgesics and repeated surgical interventions. Most recently, the use of antidepressant medications, particularly imipramine (Tofranil), has shown some good effect. Just how this works is not known, and some feel that the pain is the expression of an underlying depression which is alleviated by the antidepressant medication. In any event, it frequently is used along with psychotherapy.

The hypochondriacal patient is one of the most difficult of all. Psychotherapy is a problem with them because they do not see themselves as having any mental or emotional illness. They are convinced of the physiological aspects of their diseases and most will be seen by general practitioners and internists. The most difficult task of the physician is to remain unfrustrated and empathetic with these very unhappy and miserable people. Those working with them find the waxing and the waning of the symptoms and the chronic complaints and unhappiness very difficult to tolerate. Medication should be kept to a minimum, and every single act and drug should be explained carefully because of their suspiciousness about medications and medicine in general. Many times to expect complete cure merely insures frustration for the patient and the physician and makes the symptomatology worse.

Medications

There are no specific medications for the Somatoform Disorders except antianxiety drugs, antidepressant drugs, and analgesics. Great care must be taken with these medications due to these patients' propensity to misuse drugs. The use of the antidepressant medications in the Psychogenic Pain Disorder is the only specific pharmacological agent for this group. The other drugs are used strictly for symptomatic control; nothing more should be expected of them. Exceptionally, a hypochondriacal patient may need an antipsychotic drug when the symptoms become unbearable or when they are making life too miserable for those around them. Again, the dose should be kept as low as possible and the drug used as briefly as possible.

Other Modalities

Hypnosis, either chemically or by passive means, may be of valuable use in the Conversion Reaction, and it should be used as soon as possible. The symptoms usually respond to suggestion quickly, but this is less true of the other Somatoform Disorders. The use of hypnosis in psychogenic pain also has shown benefit in motivated patients. Experienced medical hypnotists may be able to teach the patient self-hypnosis so that minutes or even hours of relief can be produced when it is for the patient's benefit. The school teacher mentioned previously was taught self-hypnosis and could reduce the level of his pain by at least 90% for three to four hours at a time when it was necessary for him to concentrate on his work. Hypochondriacal patients rarely respond to hypnosis, and if response occurs new sensations and/or illnesses are apt to develop. The lack of trust they have in the physician and the great internal need for the symptomatology seems to prevent the beneficial effects of this treatment.

BIBLIOGRAPHY

Kenyon, F.: Hypochondriacal states. *Br. J. Psychiatry, 129:*1, 1976.

Lipsitt, D.: Medical and psychological characteristics of "crocks." *Psychiatry Med., 1:*15-25, 1970.

Pace, J.: Psychophysiology of pain: diagnostic and therapeutic implications. *J. Fam. Prac., 5:*553, 1977.

Stevens, H.: Conversion hysteria: a neurologic emergency. *Mayo Clinic Proceedings, 43:*54-64, 1968.

Wittkower, E., and Warnes, H. (eds.): *Psychosomatic Medicine: Its Clinical Application.* New York, Harper & Row, 1977.

XIII

Dissociative Disorders

This fascinating group of disorders refers to conditions in which portions of the Ego (reality testing and sense of self) are split off from or dissociated from consciousness. There is an alteration, usually sudden and temporary, in the normal functions of awareness, identity, and/or motor behavior. Whichever of these elements primarily is involved determines the specific diagnostic category.

These conditions have received much attention in literature and the entertainment media because of their dramatic qualities. Books and movies such as *The Three Faces of Eve* and *Sybil* have dramatized the multiple personality. Some form of mild, transient depersonalization, insignificant in everyday living, probably has occurred to most young adults. There have been temporary alterations in the perception of or in the experience of oneself, or a feeling of suddenly being lost or confused. Even amnesia is not too difficult to understand if one can imagine how effective this mechanism can be to reduce anxiety and to remake an unacceptable reality.

DIAGNOSTIC CATEGORIES

Psychogenic Amnesia

The major characteristic is the inability to recall important personal information when it is too great to be due to ordinary forgetfulness and is not due to some Organic Mental Disorder. Amnesia does not include conditions in which a person moves to another place and assumes a new identity; that will be discussed as Psychogenic Fugue.

There are four types of Psychogenic Amnesia.

1. Localized: A failure to remember all events occurring during a localized period of time, such as the first few hours following some stressful situation. It is not unusual for the survivor of an accident which has been fatal to a friend or relative to recall nothing that happened during the event and for the next day or two. This is the most common type of amnesia.
2. Selective Amnesia: A failure to recall some, but not all, of the events occurring during a specific period of time. The survivor mentioned above might recall making immediate hospitalization arrangements, but have no other memory of any discussion or contacts with other people around that time period.
3. Generalized Amnesia: A failure to recall all of the events of the individual's entire life (rare).
4. Continuous Amnesia: Same symptoms as Generalized Amnesia with the addition of an inability to recall even events occurring in the present (rare).

The amnesias are restricted mostly to young adults, are uncommon in middle-aged people, and rare in the elderly. They usually begin suddenly following some form of stress or prolonged boredom, and termination is equally abrupt with a good prognosis as to future recurrences. They rarely occur in happy, well adjusted people unless the stress is extraordinarily severe.

The condition must be differentiated from those similar situations produced by substance-induced intoxication, abuse of alcohol, head trauma, some types of epilepsy, and vascular disorders.

Diagnostic Criteria for Psychogenic Amnesia

A. Sudden inability to recall important personal information that is too extensive to be explained by ordinary forgetfulness.
B. The disturbance is not due to an Organic Mental Disorder.

Psychogenic Fugue

This condition is characterized by three factors: unexpected travel away from the usual locale, the assumption of a new identity, and an inability to recall the previous identity. After recovery, the individual has no recollection of the events that took place during the fugue. A person interacting with someone in a fugue state might have no idea that the individual was acting abnormally in any way.

During the illness, many fugue victims assume identities which are quite contrary to the usual personality. A shy, very unassuming and passive individual may take up a new residence and become an outgoing, apparently well integrated, aggressive person. Psychologically it appears to be a way of getting around one's Superego (internal inhibitions) and living out urges and desires that previously were repressed.

Case Example

A 35-year-old minister awakened in a hotel room in an Eastern city 500 miles from his small hometown. He was in bed with a strange woman–something absolutely foreign to his normal existence. He found that he had registered in the hotel under the name of a brother, a man who would have been quite capable of the acts which the minister had performed. The minister had no memory of having left the small town of his pastorate, but later discovered that he had been traveling under the assumed name of his brother for approximately one week. He recovered without complications except for considerable shame and guilt over his unacceptable behavior!

Fugue reactions have been known to occur for only minutes, but some have been reported to last more than a year. Recovery is expected, and although recurrences are rare, they are possible if unusual stress in the future cannot be avoided. The stress does not have to be dramatic or traumatic. It can be a life-style that is boring and dull or one which does not allow the sublimation of hostile or sexual feelings. The condition ordinarily is not difficult to differentiate from temporal lobe epilepsy, and there is no history of head trauma.

Diagnostic Criteria for Psychogenic Fugue

A. Sudden, unexpected travel from one's customary place of work or residence with inability to recall one's past.

B. Assumption of a new identity
C. No Organic Mental Disorder

Multiple Personality

This, the most dramatic of all these conditions, is characterized by the existence of two or more distinct personalities, each of which is dominant at a particular time. Each personality can have a fully integrated complex set of memories, behavioral patterns and social relationships, and transition from one personality to the other can be instantaneous, especially under stress. The original personality usually has no awareness of the other personalities, but when there are two or more subpersonalities in one person, each of them is aware of the other to some degree. This makes for a very perplexing situation, as you can imagine. One personality may interact verbally with another, and/or one personality may "listen in" to interactions between others when there are more than two.

The original personality, and even most of the subpersonalities, will be aware of periods of time for which there is no memory or only a vague one, but the patient (the true personality) rarely will volunteer this information unless questioned about it. Not infrequently the personalities are violently opposed to each other.

Case Example

A 24-year-old secretary named Janet was an extremely quiet, shy, inhibited, religious, and highly moralistic young lady. Periodically she became Jan, a flamboyant, highly sexualized, outgoing "bar hopper." Jan could speak freely and very critically of Janet, but Janet had no conscious knowledge whatsoever of Jan and her activities. Janet obviously knew that she could not account for many of her evenings, but she came to treatment only after Jan was arrested in a bar brawl and placed in the city jail. Janet found herself in jail the next morning and no longer could deny that something was wrong.

Psychosocial stress most often precipitates the transition from one personality to another, but the stress can be as undramatic as living a boring, unsatisfying life with no obvious hope of change. The transitions are very dramatic, and some of these people have been dangerous.

Case Example

One young veteran of the Korean War, originally a very passive, quiet, peaceful individual, had a very disruptive marital life. His wife had been unfaithful to him on several occasions when he was in Korea and taunted him about his lack of manliness. After one of these episodes, he dissociated into a very violent person and was arrested for severe assault on a stranger. When he was hospitalized, it was discovered that his two personalities had been present for years. Interestingly, at no time did he assault his wife and she thought his outbursts were only "temper."

It is important to differentiate Multiple Personality from the Psychotic Disorders and some types of epilepsy, but this usually is not difficult. The major personality most frequently is fairly well adapted and functioning at a level that cannot possibly be confused with psychosis.

Diagnostic Criteria for Multiple Personality

A. Existence within the same person of two or more distinct personalities, each of which is dominant at a given time.
B. The dominant personality at any particular time completely determines the individual's behavior.
C. Each personality is a complex and integrated unit with its own patterns of behavior and social relationships.

Depersonalization Disorder

Depersonalization is a less severe example of dissociation which is manifested by feeling unreal or feeling that one is not oneself. This can produce great subjective discomfort as can be imagined by looking at oneself in a mirror and seeing the reflection of a stranger. An occasional fleeting episode of something less severe than this may happen to otherwise healthy persons when under stress or fatigued, and the diagnosis should not be made unless there have been multiple episodes. Some people include somnambulism (sleepwalking) as a minor manifestation of this condition, but this is questionable. The onset of depersonalization is rapid, but it usually disappears more gradually. The term, "derealization," a situation sometimes present in Depersonalization Disorder, refers to a strange alteration in the perception of one's surroundings so that one feels that the reality of the external world is changed or lost. Objects may change size or shape and people around the patient may be perceived as dead or as robots. These patients frequently feel as if they are going insane and have many other neurotic difficulties once the depersonalization occurs. The difference between derealization and simple depersonalization is whether one changes oneself (depersonalization) or one changes the surroundings (derealization). Depersonalization is usually seen in younger people and rarely occurs after 40. Unlike the other Dissociative Disorders, there is a more frequent incidence of recurrences, although they may be mild and cause less concern than the first one.

Diagnostic Criteria for Depersonalization Disorder

A. One or more episodes of depersonalization sufficient to produce significant impairment of social or occupational functioning.
B. The symptom must not be due to any other disorder such as Schizophrenia, depression, severe anxiety, epilepsy, or an organic condition. This requires a thorough diagnostic workup.

Atypical Dissociative Disorder

Again our old friend, "atypical," is used to include those conditions in which there is a Dissociative Disorder, but in which the symptoms are not sufficient to place them in a specific category. This can include temporary trance-like states, periods of brief derealization, and strange feelings that may occur after sensory deprivation, sleep deprivation, or prolonged periods of fear or fatigue.

TREATMENT

Psychotherapy

People with Dissociative Disorders usually are extremely distressed once they become aware of these conditions. Some form of psychotherapy is essential even if recurrence is not expected, as with amnesia. Exploring alternative life-styles is worthwhile, especially when boredom and stress are involved. The patient's behavior during a fugue state or a personality dissociation may have produced unacceptable feelings of guilt, shame, or fear which need attention. For example, the preacher with the Psychogenic Fugue needed help to overcome his guilt and to accept his actions as illness rather than as sin and weakness. Multiple personalities usually require long and expert psychoanalytically-oriented psychotherapy.

Medications

Rarely are medications indicated, and none are specific.

Hypnosis

Hypnosis can be a useful tool. It is particularly helpful in an acute episode of Psychogenic Amnesia if one needs to establish the true identity rapidly. It also can be useful in the treatment phase of Multiple Personality in helping the individual "remember" and come to grips with reality factors. It was used on Janet early in treatment. She had no memory of Jan's behavior, and even though she was warned that some of these things she learned might make her uncomfortable, learning about them became an obsession. Under hypnosis she was able to remember Jan's activities, and this aided her to understand the parts of her personality that had led her to this dissociation. The end product was a Janet with some of Jan's better qualities, but with them under control and more socially acceptable.

Depersonalization Disorder responds to psychotherapy alone in most instances, and again one concentrates upon the reality factors which might lead the individual to need to dissociate from real life. That, in fact, is the basis of most of the psychotherapeutic work. Many of these conditions stem from lives which are boring, frustrating, and unhappy, but from which there appears to be no escape.

BIBLIOGRAPHY

Balis, J., Wurmser, L., and McDaniel, E. (eds.): *Clinical Psychopathology,* pp. 207-330, Boston, Butterworth, 1978.

Cattell, J.: Depersonalization Phenomena. In *American Handbook of Psychiatry,* S. Arieti (ed.), New York, Basic Books, 1966.

Kiersch, T.: Amnesia: a clinical study of 98 cases. *Am. J. Psychiatry, 119:*57-60, 1962.

Ludwig, A., Brandsma, J., Wilber, C., Bendfeldt, F., and Jameson, D.: The objective study of a multiple personality. *Arch. Gen. Psychiatry, 26:*298-310, 1972.

Thigpen, C., and Cleckley, H.: *The Three Faces of Eve.* New York, McGraw-Hill, 1957.

XIV

Psychosexual Disorders

This group of disorders specifically means that there is a sexual dysfunction that is caused, or assumed to be caused, by psychological factors. Aberrations of sexual functioning have fascinated writers throughout history, and many of the best descriptions of them have been done by people like the Marquis de Sade, who was afflicted with more than one paraphilia. They are divided into four major groups:

1. The Gender Identity Disorders
2. The Paraphilias
3. Psychosexual Dysfunctions
4. Other Psychosexual Disorders

There are subdivisions of these major categories and each has its own special fascination and characteristics.

A word of caution: Sexual dysfunction is a popular topic for humor and a constant target for strong feelings and prejudices. It has been connected throughout history with misunderstanding, bias, ignorance, persecution, and downright cruelty. Some of the disorders are relatively unimportant, but many of them are of extreme personal and social significance. All should be taken seriously. They are illnesses, not sins or disgraces.

THE GENDER IDENTITY DISORDERS

Gender identity is the sense of knowing to which sex one belongs. Most people are fully aware, without question, that they are either male or female, and this awareness is congruent with the external genitalia. A disturbance in gender identity, in the sense of maleness or femaleness, is rare and must not be confused with very common feelings of inadequacy in fulfilling one's gender role. Gender role refers to the public expression of one's gender identity, not to the feeling of maleness or femaleness.

Transsexualism

The transsexual individual possesses the internal and external genitalia, the chromosomes, and the hormones of one sex, but the psychic apparatus of the other. The core gender identity is developed in direct contradiction to the anatomy, and there is much evidence that core gender identity is established firmly before 2-1/2 years of age. The diagnosis is made only if the disturbance has been continuous for at least two years and is due to no other mental disorder. These unfortunate people are uncomfortable wearing the clothes of their anatomic sex, and frequently they find their genitals repugnant, almost as if they were tumorous growths. Some males may cross-dress, take female hormones, have beards removed, and pass relatively indistinguishable from normal females.

Most true transsexuals have evident gender identity problems as children, but some do not become aware of their condition until late adolescence or early adulthood. They frequently present to physicians with requests that their genitalia be removed. Anatomical males have the condition more commonly than females, although it is possible that females do not present with this complaint as often as males due to the greater difficulty of surgical treatment. The condition must be distinguished from Homosexuality, but that usually is not difficult. The homosexual male does not wish to have his penis amputated!

The cause is not understood fully. It is known that many of these children have received strong messages from birth that they were members of the other sex or that the family expected them to be and to act as if they were. Signals, such as name, dress, play, were given to contradict the anatomical sex.

Diagnostic Criteria for Transsexualism

A. Pervasive sense that one's anatomical sex is inappropriate and opposite to the true self.
B. Wish to be rid of one's genitals and to live as a member of the other sex.
C. The disturbance has been continuous (not limited to stress periods) for at least two years.
D. The absence of physical intersexual or genetic abnormalities and due to no other physical or mental illness.

Gender Identity Disorder of Childhood

These children persistently feel uncomfortable and inappropriate about their anatomic sex and may insist that they belong to the other gender. This must not be confused with mere "tomboyishness" in girls or "sissified behavior" in boys. They tend to avoid playing with individuals of their own sex and may claim that they will grow up to be members of the opposite sex. The boys prefer dressing in girls' clothing and using female toys, and the reverse is true of the girls. This usually begins before the fourth birthday, and there are social consequences in that the peers begin to ostracize these children, to make fun of them, and to make normal friendships and peer group relations more difficult.

The predisposing factors are felt to be difficulties in the parent-infant relationship. The mothers have encouraged an excessive and prolonged closeness with the sons, and it appears that the girls have either too closely identified with the father or have been pushed away from identification with the mother for some reason or other including illnesses, separations, or psychological factors.

Diagnostic Criteria for Gender Identity Disorder of Childhood

For females:

A. Strongly stated desire to be a boy or insistence that she is a boy.

B. Persistent denial of female anatomy as manifested by at least one of the following beliefs:
   1. She will grow up to become a man.
   2. She will not become pregnant.
   3. She will not develop breasts.
   4. She has no vagina.
   5. That she has, or will have, a penis.

C. Onset of disturbance before puberty.

For males:

A. Strong persistent desire to be a girl or insistence that he is a girl.

B. Either:
   1. Persistent repudiation of male genitals by repeated assurances that he will grow up to become a woman, that his penis or testes are disgusting and will disappear, and that it would be better not to have a penis.
   2. Preoccupation with female activities as manifested by either cross-dressing or by a compelling desire to participate in the pastimes of girls.

C. Onset of disturbance before puberty.

Treatment of Gender Identity Disorders

The treatment of Transsexualism is a controversial issue. These unfortunate people do not wish to have their feelings altered; they want their bodies changed. Many of them have personality disorders, something that seems quite logical in view of the misery of their existences. Psychotherapy may help the person adjust to the reality of the situation, but it will not reverse the basic pathology.

Surgery has been more successful for the anatomical males than for the females. It is possible to remove the male genitalia and to create a workable vagina and to produce reasonable breasts with female hormones. It is not possible to create a workable set of male genitals for the transsexual female. Many of these women are satisfied to have the breasts and uteri removed and to receive male hormones to give them a more masculine voice and face.

Most clinics involved in transsexual surgery have insisted upon at least a year's cross-dressing and psychotherapy combined with hormonal therapy before attempting irreversible surgery. This is a prolonged and expensive procedure which involves many legal and social parameters such as changes in draft status, driver's license, birth certificate, social security, and it is obvious that a lawyer must be consulted. The extreme difficulties, the uncertain outcome, and the enormous expense has led to a recent decline in the use of surgical treatment.

The Gender Identity Disorder of Childhood needs immediate attention. Family intervention before the condition becomes fixed may be successful, but it requires the cooperation of both parents and child. These youngsters must be helped to obtain a proper identification figure and to receive approval from the parenting figures for acting in the appropriate sexual manner. The earlier the intervention is begun, the better is the prognosis, and once the child reaches adolescence the incidence of Homosexuality and Transvestism (to be discussed later) increases, and the chance of change decreases.

PARAPHILIAS

This group of disorders previously was called "sexual deviations." This term indicated that the process of sexual maturation had deviated from the norm in relationship to the sexual object, sexual aim, or sexual drive. The essential feature of the Paraphilias is that unusual or bizarre imagery or acts are essential for sexual excitement. Such imagery or acts are insistent, involuntary, repetitive, and generally involve:

1. Preference for nonhuman objects for sexual arousal,
2. Repetitive sexual activity with humans involving real or simulated suffering or humiliation or,
3. Repetitive sexual activity with nonconsenting partners.

There are all degrees and varieties of sexual activity in this world, and the social norm of one group may appear abnormal to another. Some acts, such as mild bondage, may be playful and harmless with a consenting partner, but if carried to an extreme degree it may be injurious and become sadistic and masochistic. Many of these conditions are complicated by the fact that they also are illegal and, in many instances, totally socially unacceptable.

The mechanism of denial is a major feature in the Paraphilias. Most of these people do not think their behavior is abnormal and do not see themselves as ill. Some will admit to guilt and shame and depression, but this usually follows being caught in the act or some legal or social coercion. The social and sexual relationships of people with paraphilias may be abnormal, and the people with these conditions tend to be underachievers and immature in nonsexual areas of living.

The specific disorders are:

Fetishism

The characteristic of Fetishism is the use of inanimate objects (fetishes) as the preferred or exclusive method of achieving sexual excitement. The diagnosis is not made when the fetish is limited to some article of female clothing used in cross-dressing, or when it is used as a stimulus to heterosexual behavior. The fetishistic object is endowed with sexual significance which allows the person (usually a male) to avoid contact with the female. Objects of female clothing are most commonly used, and the usual behavior is for the male to use the object as an aid to masturbation. The fetish ordinarily is used only one time, and most fetishistic objects must be obtained surreptitiously. For example, a man with a shoe fetish would not get a sexual charge out of a shoe which he bought in a clothing store. He would need to take it from some female, preferably one he knew. Incidentally, shoes and feet have been endowed with sexual significance since biblical times and for many centuries the Chinese made mutilation of female feet a social norm for sexual attractiveness.

The disorder almost always begins in early adolescence and tends to be chronic. Most of these males are immature in many other ways and tend to be called "loners" by their peers and family.

Diagnostic Criteria for Fetishism

A. The use of non-living objects (fetishes) as the preferred or exclusive method of achieving sexual excitement.

B. The objects are not limited to articles of female clothing used in cross-dressing or to objects designed to be used for stimulation to heterosexual intercourse.

Transvestism

Transvestism is dressing in the clothing of the opposite sex in order to become erotically aroused. It ranges from the man who occasionally wears some single piece of female clothing to the one who cross-dresses totally and appears to adapt himself to all female mannerisms possible. Most of these people (mostly men) are heterosexual, and many use a cross-dressing episode as a prelude to intercouse.

Case Example

A television executive with four children after 16 years of marriage was hospitalized for a Depressive Disorder. He told of his life-long need to dress in his wife's brassiere and panties before being able to consummate sexual intercourse. He would put on these articles of clothing, admire himself in the mirror or have his wife admire him, then take off the clothing and engage in heterosexual intercourse. Neither his wife nor the man was concerned about what they considered a mild eccentricity that did not interfere with daily living.

Cross-dressing usually begins in childhood or early adolescence, but may not be done in public until adulthood. There may be one particular article of clothing that is erotic, but most transvestites also need to be admired by someone else or to admire themselves in a mirror. These men commonly give a history of having been punished or humiliated in childhood by the parents forcing them to dress in the clothing of girls.

Case Example

One transvestite vividly remembered that he had been a constant bedwetter until his early teens. His mother had made him wear his sister's clothing and walk in front of their house in full view of his peers each time he had wet the bed, which was almost daily.

> This had occurred from his earliest memory in grammar school. He first succumbed to an irresistible urge to wear women's clothing when he was a senior in high school. Without wearing some article of female outer clothing, he was impotent.

Psychodynamically there is a peculiar situation in which the male truly feels that it is the female who is the strong, penis-bearing individual. It appears that in the unconscious the donning of female clothing allows this man to act truly masculine, a characteristic he attributes to the female. The transvestite's mother usually has been the dominant figure in the family. The condition, except for the social overtones of it, is harmless.

Diagnostic Criteria for Transvestism

A. Recurrent and persistent cross-dressing by a heterosexual male.
B. Use of cross-dressing for the purpose of sexual excitement.
C. Intense frustration when the cross-dressing is impossible.
D. Does not meet the criteria for Transsexualism.

Zoophilia

Zoophilia, sometimes called bestiality, is the condition in which the use of animals is the preferred or exclusive method of achieving sexual excitement. It usually is a farm animal or a pet, and the condition has no legal or damaging consequences other than whatever it may indicate about the personality of the individual. It indicates that these people have difficulty in relating to humans, and they will tend to be underachieving, passive, semi-withdrawn people. An isolated act of Zoophilia is not rare in adolescence among such people as farm boys and sheep herders, but the diagnosis is made only when it persists as a preferred or exclusive method of achieving sexual excitement.

Diagnostic Criteria for Zoophilia

A. The act or fantasy of engaging in sexual activity with animals as a repeated or exclusive method of achieving sexual excitement.

Pedophilia

Pedophilia is a serious disorder both socially and legally. It refers to the individual, almost always male, who engages in sexual activity with prepubertal children as the preferred or exclusive method of achieving sexual excitement. There is great variation in this condition from the man who makes no sexual advances to children, but who finds himself much more comfortable relating to them, to the male who is totally impotent except with children. The condition can be heterosexual or homosexual, and when it is homosexual, it indicates a more deeply-seated pathology. Homosexually oriented males tend to prefer slightly older children, whereas heterosexually oriented pedophiles prefer eight- to ten-year-old girls, although this is variable. Actual sexual intercourse with the victims of pedophiles is uncommon. The preferred sexual activity mostly is limited to looking and/or touching. Most of these men who are heterosexually oriented are married, but that is not true of the homosexual group.

The condition usually begins in late teens or early adulthood, but it may not occur until middle or later age. When it occurs for the first time in an elderly individual, some form of Organic Brain Syndrome should be suspected, and the condition may be only one indication of a more generalized regression to childish activities.

The pedophiliac male fears sexual contact with an adult and acts toward the child as he wishes his parents had acted toward him. Many will say that they would be humiliated to approach an adult female, and almost all profess a great love and respect for children. The heterosexual pedophile rarely hurts the child physically, and even though the homosexual pedophile is more apt to resort to some form of violence, this is not common. The condition tends to be very upsetting to a family and a community, and one of the most important aspects of it is the treatment of the pedophile's victim. It is important that the child not be made to feel that something horrible has happened and, above all, the situation should be handled calmly, cooly, and with as little publicity as possible.

Diagnostic Criteria for Pedophilia

A. The act or fantasy of engaging in sexual activity with prepubertal children as a repeatedly preferred or exclusive method of achieving sexual excitement.

B. In adults, the prepubertal children are at least ten years younger than the individual, but this age difference is not required and clinical judgment must be taken into account when dealing with an adolescent.

Exhibitionism

Exhibitionism probably is the most prevalent of the Paraphilias, and it is one most often repeated. It is the repetitive act of exposing the genitals to an unsuspecting stranger for the purpose of achieving sexual excitement, but with no attempt at further sexual activity. The exhibitionist wishes to surprise, shock, or disgust the observer in order to reassure himself that he has a powerful and dangerous organ. Some may masturbate during the exposure, others after, but many may go home and behave as normal heterosexuals.

The condition usually begins in late adolescence and peaks in the middle 20s, but tends to "burn out" for some unknown reason in later years. Arrests for Exhibitionism after age 40 are relatively uncommon.

These men usually have had mothers who have been the powerful figures in the family, and this appears to have made it difficult for them to develop a true sense of masculine identity and self-confidence. Usually, they are heterosexual and most will be otherwise relatively normal people. They rarely expose themselves to acquaintances or in their own neighborhoods, and equally rarely do they make any great attempts to escape recognition. They do not harm the person to whom they exhibit, and the act is not an invitation to sexual intercourse. Most often the urge to exhibit occurs when something has happened to the man to lower his self-esteem or to create a feeling of anxiety.

Case Example

Mr. Pope had been arrested many times for exhibitionism and had served several jail sentences by age 35. He worked as a printer in a small city, had two children, and was an ideal church going citizen in his community. He had been in treatment (group therapy) for his exhibitionism for nine months with no difficulties. One afternoon he exhibited himself to some high school girls and was arrested. Mr. Pope had made a mistake in his work the previous day and had been embarrassed and humiliated by his employer. This blow to his self-esteem appeared to be the precipitating cause of a repeat of the exhibitionism.

Diagnostic Criteria for Exhibitionism

A. Repetitive acts of exposing the penis to an unsuspecting stranger for the purpose of achieving sexual excitement, but not for the purpose of achieving sexual activity.

Voyeurism

The opposite side of the coin from Exhibitionism is Voyeurism. These men, called "Peeping Toms," achieve sexual gratification by surreptitiously viewing a nude female or some part of her body, with or without observing any sexual activity. The man usually masturbates during the voyeuristic activity or goes home and relives what he saw in fantasy while he masturbates. Parenthetically, the term "Peeping Tom" was coined when a tailor named Tom reputedly refused to cover his eyes when Lady Godiva rode down the streets of Coventry in the nude!

It is necessary for the voyeuristic act to be forbidden and done surreptitiously. A voyeur may not enjoy a strip show or a burlesque performance and many even find it disgusting. Voyeurism represents "rape with the eyes," and you will recall that our society does give the eyes a great deal of magical power. We speak of the "evil eye," "undressing with the eyes," and certain societies feel that thoughts can be read through the eyes.

The onset usually is in early adulthood and one or two episodes of the activity do not necessarily lead to the chronic condition. Rarely do these individuals make any attempt to assault the viewed female, and many of them are otherwise productive, normally heterosexual people. There is an uncommon incidence of premature overexposure to nude female bodies in the backgrounds of these men.

Case Examples

A geological engineer had been arrested innumerable time for Voyeurism. He was absolutely unable to control the urges for over one to two weeks at a time. His father had died when he was four years of age and his mother had become a severe alcoholic. When he came home from school she was almost always drunk, and when so, she disrobed herself completely. For the next 15 years of his life, it had been his job to dress his nude mother almost every day and put her to bed. He began his voyeurism at age 16.

Another severe voyeur had been raised in a fatherless home with his mother and a sister one year older. It had been their habit throughout life to wear no clothing in the house and for all to use the bathroom simultaneously if so desired. He adamantly denied that this was, or ever had been, sexually arousing.

Diagnostic Criteria for Voyeurism

A. The individual repeatedly and surreptitiously observes people who are naked, in the act of disrobing, or engaging in sexual activity, but with no desire to seek sexual activity with that person.

B. The "peeping" is the repeatedly preferred or exclusive method of achieving sexual excitement.

Sexual Masochism

The essential feature of Masochism is sexual excitement produced by suffering. The diagnosis is warranted under one of two conditions:

1. The preferred or exclusive method of producing sexual excitement is to be humiliated, bound, beaten, or otherwise made to suffer.
2. The person had intentionally participated in some activity in which there was physical harm or the life was threatened in order to produce sexual excitement.

The condition usually begins in early childhood as fantasy. It tends to be chronic and have many variations from mild infliction of emotional pain to conditions which actually produce death. Many of these people have a history of being victims of physical aggression in childhood, and it appears that there has been an association of their discomfort with the sexual impulse. They tend to see sex as forbidden and evil unless atoned for by some form of suffering.

Bondage perhaps is the mildest form of true Masochism.

Case Examples

A 40-year-old physician and father of two children became less and less interested in sexual activity unless his wife would first tie him tightly to an unpadded kitchen chair after he had undressed. The ropes needed to be tight enough to produce actual pain and circulatory embarrassment and to be kept on for several minutes. His wife would untie him and normal sexual relations would proceed when he was ready.

A 32-year-old otherwise healthy female was unable to achieve orgasm until her husband had lashed her buttocks and thighs rather severely with a length of rubber hose. The condition had produced a lot of fibrous tissue on her body and, even at her early age, it was beginning to be difficult for her to sit in hard chairs. Despite this inconvenience, she continued the practice. This woman had been beaten repeatedly by her father and a stepfather in early childhood and had been seduced by a second stepfather at age 11.

Diagnostic Criteria for Sexual Masochism

There must be either:

1. A preferred or exclusive method of producing sexual excitement by being humiliated, bound, beaten, or otherwise made to suffer.
2. The intentional participation in an activity in which physical harm occurred or life was threatened in order to produce sexual excitement.

Sexual Sadism

The Frenchman, the Marquis de Sade, wrote about his own life and gave his name to this paraphilia. It is the opposite of Masochism in that it is the infliction of physical or psychological suffering on another person in order to achieve sexual excitement. The diagnosis can be made under any of three different conditions:

1. The individual has repeatedly and intentionally inflicted psychological or physical suffering on a nonconsenting partner in order to achieve sexual excitement.
2. The repeated and preferred or exclusive mode of achieving sexual excitement combines humiliation with some form of body suffering on a consenting partner.
3. Injury that is extensive, permanent, or possibly deadly is inflicted on a consenting partner in order to achieve sexual excitement.

These people usually have had sadistic fantasies since early childhood. One college freshman told of having begun to masturbate even before puberty and to imagine that he was slicing up females and flushing them down the toilet. As an adult he had become unable to be sexually aroused without first inflicting physical pain on his partner.

There can be great variation in sadistic practices from the individual who merely wishes to inflict a slight degree of humiliation to the one who mutilates and murders the victim. The backgrounds of these people frequently show an inordinate amount of brutality and a complete lack of respect for the opposite sex. Some forms of rape represent Sexual Sadism, but this does not mean that all rapists are also sadists.

Diagnostic Criteria for Sexual Sadism

One of the following:

1. The individual repeatedly, intentionally inflicts psychological or physical suffering in order to produce sexual excitement on a nonconsenting partner.

2. The repeatedly preferred or exclusive mode of achieving sexual excitement combines humiliation with simulated or mildly injurious bodily suffering on a consenting partner.
3. Bodily injury that is extensive, permanent, or even deadly is inflicted on a consenting partner in order to achieve sexual excitement.

Atypical Paraphilias

You cannot imagine an object, an act, a fantasy, or a situation which some individual has not used to produce sexual arousal. Most are of no great clinical significance because they are relatively harmless or quite rare, but they tend to produce strong feelings of disgust and aversion in most people.

Briefly described, some of them are:

1. *Coprophilia:* This represents an unusual sexualization of feces, the act of defecating, or something so related. A successful practicing physician was able to convince at least one or two women patients each week that it was a necessary part of his examination for him to watch them have a bowel movement. He would do so, masturbate after watching them, but otherwise treat them perfectly legitimately and make no sexual advances.
2. *Necrophilia:* This is a situation in which the individual is unable to relate sexually to live females. Usually, these are very borderline men who find work in funeral homes or situations which allow them to contact dead females. An interesting variation on necrophilia is an occasional male who cannot be aroused unless his sexual partner lies completely motionless during intercourse.
3. *Telephone Scatologia:* This is a form of Exhibitionism in which the individual uses words rather than the penis. The man calls an unsuspecting female, frequently chosen at random from the phone book, and attempts to engage her in extremely lewd and pornographic conversation. Rarely does he attempt to contact the woman otherwise.
4. *Urophilia:* Here the fascination is with urine and urination just as it was with feces and defecation in Coprophilia.

Case Example

A very successful middle-aged businessman made trips to a distant city about once every six months. While there he would hire a call girl at a major hotel to have dinner with him. His only request was that she hold her desire to urinate as long as possible and then give him a brief warning. They would go to his room, he would lie nude on the bathroom floor while she urinated in his face and over his body, then he paid her and again became the affluent, conservative businessman.

5. *Frotteurism:* This is a fascination with buttocks. These men usually rub against or fondle buttocks on crowded elevators, subways, and buses so that it appears to be an accidental contact.

Treatment of Paraphilias

The Paraphilias vary from extreme tragedy (Sadism) to mere annoyances (Frotteurism). Treatment is particularly difficult because the people rarely feel that they are ill (denial) and do not seek intervention. These conditions usually come to light either secondary to other illnesses or because of pressure from the neighborhood or the police. It is important to remember that, even though the act may be illegal, it is due to an emotional illness. Prison sentences do more harm than good, and enlightened courts are more apt to sentence these men to treatment centers than to jail. Enforced therapy may be the only way that some of these unfortunate individuals, mostly men, can break through their mechanism of denial.

Modalities:

1. *Group therapy:* This has proven to be effective in several of the conditions, especially Exhibitionism, Voyeurism, and Pedophilia. Fortunately, these three categories make up the largest number of offenders. The therapy usually takes from one to two years of regular attendance, but most of these men can be kept in society as functioning citizens.

2. *Medication:* Medications have little place in the treatment except in rare cases of extreme sexual violence. Research is continuing on the use of antiandrogenic hormones which allow for temporary chemical castration. There is some evidence that these men, for example: rapists and sadists, may be returned to normal masculine functioning after a year or two of chemical castration and proper group therapy.
3. *Behavioral Modification:* Various forms of aversion therapy have been used for most of these conditions. The reports of success are variable and controversial.

Perhaps the most important point is a proper assessment of the danger of the individual to the community. One should be extremely cautious when a Paraphilia is associated with two factors: a psychotic background and/or violence. In either of these conditions, treatment on an outpatient basis is a calculated risk.

The greatest treatment of all would be prevention. We may not know the exact cause of these conditions, but we know that they rarely are seen in individuals who have been raised in a stable home situation in which the parent figures demonstrated respect for the sexuality of each other and love and approval of the child in its anatomical sex role.

PSYCHOSEXUAL DYSFUNCTIONS

This group of conditions refers to an inhibition in the sexual drive and/or the inability to complete sexual intercourse successfully. This category does not apply when there is an organic dysfunction such as severe diabetes, or when the condition is due to external conditions such as alcohol or drug abuse.

First, a quick review of the normal sexual intercourse cycle.

1. Arousal: This is a psychological and physiological situation which usually begins with fantasies and then the desire to have sexual activity. It varies tremendously from person to person so that a normal 25-year-old may desire sexual intercourse one time per month whereas another equally normal person may desire it once daily. The certain sign of sexual

arousal in the male is penile erection and the counterpart of this in the female is vaginal lubrication. Many other physiological responses may occur, but these are the main ones.

2. Plateau: The arousal period merges into the plateau in which there is vasocongestion increasing in the pelvis and the vaginal areas of the female and a heightening sense of excitement and tension in the male. Many other forms of vasodilitation and autonomic nervous system activity may be evident such as nipple enlargement, flushing, rapid heart rate, and sweating.
3. Orgasm: The orgasm in the male is accompanied by ejaculatory emission, but in the female the physiological components are not as evident. There are minor contractions of the uterus and the outer third of the vagina, but in both male and female there may be involuntary muscular activities of any part of the body.
4. Resolution: This usually consists of a sense of relaxation and well being and is accompanied by a return of the vascular system to normal. The male undergoes resolution much more rapidly than the female, and usually cannot return to the arousal phase for some period of time.

Problems can occur in any one of these four areas. They may be primary, having always been present, or they may be secondary, having occurred in what once was a satisfactory sexual response. The fact that an individual does not have sexual desire should not be taken as a pathological sign unless that individual is unhappy about it. One must keep constantly in mind the tremendous variation in the sexual lives of human beings and not fall prey to biases and stereotypes from the literature.

Diagnostic Categories

Inhibited Sexual Desire

Diagnostic Criteria

A. Persistent and pervasive inhibition of sexual desire. One must consider such factors as health, age, previous sexual activities, and the total context of the person's life. This complaint usually means that there is a source of distress in either the person or the partner.

B. The disturbance is not caused exclusively by organic factors or medications.

Inhibited Sexual Excitement

This designation replaces the old terms, frigidity and impotence.

Diagnostic Criteria

A. Recurrent and persistent inhibition of sexual excitement during sexual activity manifested in males by partial or complete failure to attain or maintain erection until completion of the sexual act. In females, there is partial or complete failure to attain or maintain the lubrication-sexual excitement response until completion of the sexual act.

B. The clinical judgment that the individual is engaging in sexual activity that is adequate in focus, intensity, and duration.

C. The disturbance is not caused by organic factors or medication.

A word is in order here about the changing incidence. Impotence, or Inhibited Sexual Excitement, among young males was rare until recently. Clinicians now are seeing a great amount of what is called "performance anxiety" as the major cause for Inhibited Sexual Excitement, and this may occur even in the late teens. On the other hand, this condition has become less common among females as sexuality has emerged from the Victorian Period and has become much more acceptable. The condition is a very disturbing one for which many people seek help.

Inhibited Female Orgasm

Diagnostic Criteria

A. Recurrent and persistent inhibition of the female orgasm following a normal sexual excitement phase. There may or may not be a difficulty of inhibition with the sexual excitement. Some women may have orgasm under specific conditions, such as manual stimulation of the clitoris. The evaluation of this condition requires a complete knowledge of the woman's sexual life and personality.

B. The disturbance is not caused by organic factors or medication.

Inhibited Male Orgasm

Diagnostic Criteria

A. Recurrent and persistent inhibition of orgasm as manifested by delay or absence of ejaculation following adequate sexual stimulation and excitement.

B. Not caused by organic factors or medications.

Premature Ejaculation

Diagnostic Criteria

A. Ejaculation occurring before the individual wishes it because of persistent absence of reasonable voluntary control during sexual activity. This judgment of "reasonable control" must be made by considering the factors that affect duration of the excitement phase such as age, partner, preliminary activity, setting, etc.

B. The disturbance is not due to a known condition.

Functional Dyspareunia

Dyspareunia means painful intercourse and the patient will be female over 95% of the time. This diagnosis must never be made until all physical reasons for the pain have been ruled out beyond doubt.

Diagnostic Criteria

A. Intercourse associated with recurrent and persistent genital pain in either the male or the female, but rarely seen in the male.

B. The disturbance must not be caused by physical disorder, vaginismus, or other conditions.

Functional Vaginismus

The uncontrollable spasms of the perineal muscles is the patient's way of preventing the insertion of the penis, even when it is consciously desired. The unconscious component, as in Dyspareunia, is a fear of the male penis which symbolizes possible pain and damage.

Diagnostic Criteria

A. Recurrent history of involuntary spasm of the musculature of the outer third of the vagina so as to interfere with intercourse.

B. No physical disorder to account for the above.

Treatment of Psychosexual Dysfunctions

No Psychosexual Dysfunction should be diagnosed or treated without a comprehensive physical, laboratory, and psychiatric examination of the individual. In most instances, this should include the sexual partner. Experienced researchers and clinicians have time and again discovered that the sexual dysfunctions rarely exist alone. There usually is some other psychopathology, although not necessarily severe, or there is a relationship difficulty between the people involved. To concentrate on the dysfunction alone is bad medicine.

A definitive description of the treatment of these conditions is not within the scope of this book, but the works of Masters and Johnson and Helen Kaplan are superb references for those who wish to go more deeply into the subject. This will deal only with generalities and will assume that all organic factors have been ruled out. The general aim of the treatment is to maximize pleasure, relaxation, and intimacy and to minimize guilt, tensions, and anxieties. After the complete workup of the couple, the evaluation considers:

1. Psychopathology in either partner
2. The quality of the relationship
3. The role the sexual symptoms play in the relationship and the intrapsychic dynamics of the couple.

Treatment results will be best when both partners are emotionally healthy and is contraindicated when either partner is psychotic, severely depressed, or actively paranoid. Neurotic individuals may respond well if one understands their defenses and respects them.

Fortunately, the most frequent cause is a relatively superficial anxiety such as anticipation of failure. If only this is true and the people have respect and affection for each other, the prognosis is good. When there are deep-seated fears of intimacy or there is a hostile relationship, the prognosis is bad.

Although there are specific treatments for each of the conditions listed, they all include some degree of what is known as "sensate focusing" or "pleasuring." These are graded steps by which the individuals learn to desensitize themselves to the anxieties while maximizing the pleasure of touch and of intimacy. In certain specific conditions such as Vaginismus, forms of desensitization by gradual dilatation of the vagina, combined with pleasuring exercises are very effective.

OTHER PSYCHOSEXUAL DISORDERS

Homosexuality

The homosexual person is one who habitually and by choice obtains sexual gratification from persons of the same sex. By definition, this excludes an individual, commonly a pre-adolescent or adolescent, who has had only a sexual experimentation with a member of the same sex. It also excludes sexual acts which may occur under deprived situations such as in prisons. The American Psychiatric Association has determined that the condition of Homosexuality does not, by itself, constitute an illness. It is listed as a disorder only when the individual finds the behavior repugnant or inconsistent with his or her basic desires.

Homosexuality is not a normal biological situation. Removing the condition from the class of illnesses came about for two reasons. First: many, perhaps even the majority, of homosexual people function well within the normal emotional and mental range.

Second: classifying all homosexuals as ill was a social injustice added to an already difficult and sometimes very persecuted life-style.

The development of heterosexual identification is at once very simple and extremely complex. The simple aspect is that it occurs from the identification with and the desire to be like the parent of the same sex and to choose as a love object someone similar to the parent of the opposite sex. The complexity is that there are many variations and subtleties which can lead to incomplete and insecure sexual identification.

A variety of conditions may make proper identification difficult. There may be no same-sexed parent after whom to model oneself, or that parent may be unattractive or even repugnant. The parent of the opposite sex may be overly seductive and may communicate to the child that functioning sexually in accordance with anatomic sex will lead to disapproval. An overseductive mother may produce a young man who so identifies with her that he becomes feminine in his gender role. The opposite may be true of a female child whose father forms a more attractive identification figure than the mother. The most important aspect in the development of mature heterosexuality is for the child to be raised by parents who are well adjusted in their sexual roles and who approve of the child as a functioning male or female.

Ego-dystonic Homosexuality

This diagnosis is made when an individual does not like being homosexual and/or wishes to become heterosexual because the condition is unwanted and a persistent source of distress. These people ordinarily have found their homosexual relationships unsatisfactory and accompanied by emotional upset with feelings of shame, guilt, and/or disgust. Loneliness and a sense of isolation and depression usually are present. The individual ordinarily becomes aware of this in early adolescence after negative feelings about homosexuality already have developed.

Most homosexual people give up wanting to become heterosexual and accept themselves eventually. This is particularly true when there is a supportive homosexual subculture and when the individual discovers that the change to heterosexuality may be a long, arduous, and frequently unsuccessful project.

Most homosexuals realize that they are at a distinct disadvantage in a heterosexual society. Even in our much more open and enlightened society, homosexuality is not accepted by most people. Their lives are filled with conflict in society, fears over employment, and in many instances they are the butts of jokes and actual persecution. This means that the well adjusted homosexual has to develop Ego Defense Mechanisms to reconcile himself with the greater society since approximately 90% to 95% of the world is heterosexual.

Diagnostic Criteria for Ego-dystonic Homosexuality

A. The individual persistently is without heterosexual arousal and is unhappy that this significantly interferes with initiating or maintaining wanted heterosexual relationships.
B. There is a sustained pattern of homosexual arousal that the individual explicitly states is a persistent source of unwanted distress.

Treatment of Ego-dystonic Homosexuality

Treatment first consists of a thorough evaluation of the individual's degree of homosexuality. This is done by an assessment of the entire past history with a determination of heterosexual components of the personality. Are the dreams heterosexual or homosexual? What are the masturbatory fantasies? Can or has the individual ever been aroused by the opposite sex? Does the individual find a fantasy of sexual contact with the opposite sex pleasant or disgusting? No matter how ego-dystonic the situation might be, the individual who has no heterosexual characteristics has little chance of becoming converted. Treatment will consist of psychotherapy aimed at helping this person adjust to the homosexual condition and to live as fully as possible.

The more the heterosexual indications and the more dystonic the homosexual life, the more it may be possible for the individual to respond to prolonged psychoanalytically oriented psychotherapy.

Behavioral modification techniques have been used with some reported success, but this is a controversial issue. These techniques include situations in which the individual is made uncomfortable with homosexual stimuli, and since they are very varied and complex, the reader is referred to references for more detail.

BIBLIOGRAPHY

Kaplan, H.: *The Illustrated Manual of Sex Therapy.* New York, Quadrangle/ The New York Times Book Co., 1975.

Kolodny, R., Masters, W., and Johnson, V.: The Paraphilias. In *Textbook of Sexual Medicine,* pp. 575-586. Boston, Little, Brown and Co., 1979.

Masters, W., and Johnson, V.: *Human Sexual Inadequacy.* Boston, Little, Brown and Co., 1970.

Mathis, J.: *Clear Thinking About Sexual Deviations.* Chicago, Nelson-Hall Co., 1972.

Mohr, J., Turner, R., and Jerry, M.: *Pedophilia and Exhibitionism.* Toronto, U. of Toronto Press, 1964.

Saghir, M., and Robins, E.: *Male and Female Homosexuality.* Baltimore, Williams and Wilkins, 1973.

Stoller, R.: *Perversion.* New York, Pantheon Books, 1975.

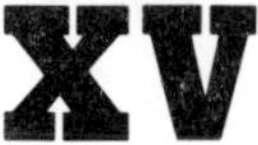

Factitious Disorders

"Factitious" means not genuine, not factual. These disorders are characterized by physical or psychological symptoms produced by the individual and under voluntary control, but one must modify the usual understanding of "voluntary control." The sense of voluntary control is subjective, and is inferred only by the outside observer. These acts have a compulsive quality in the sense that the patient is unable to prevent the behavior even when its self-destructive aspect is recognized. The actions are considered "voluntary" only in the sense that they are deliberate and purposeful, but not in the sense that they actually can be controlled by the patient's will power. They are voluntary acts used to pursue involuntarily (unconscious) adopted goals.

Factitious Disorders must be distinguished from Malingering. The malingering patient also is in voluntary control of the symptoms, but the behavior has a goal which can be identified rather than one which exists for psychological reasons alone. If a man simulates a mental or a physical illness in order to get out of dangerous military duty, that is voluntary (conscious) and has a recognizable goal, therefore it is Malingering, not a Factitious Disorder. The only goal of the true Factitious Disorder is to assume the role of a patient; it always implies psychopathology and a very severe personality disturbance. In the past many of these people were classified as severe hysterics.

FACTITIOUS DISORDER WITH PSYCHOLOGICAL SYMPTOMS

The essential feature is the voluntary production of severe psychological symptoms suggestive of mental disorder, most often a psychosis. The main goal is to assume the role of a patient, and if there is other recognizable gain, it is coincidental. This condition has been called Ganser's syndrome, pseudopsychosis, and pseudodementia.

It is characterized by a complex of psychological symptoms that invariably are presented or become worse when the patient is being observed and may be absent when the patient is alone. There can be any known mental symptoms from amnesia to a variety of hallucinations and strange somatic reactions. The patients vary from being extremely suggestible to being totally negative, and many of their symptoms appear to be "silly." For example, a patient asked how many legs are on a chair standing nearby may point to it and say, "three." Asked to multiply 6 x 6, the patient may say, "37." The answer will approximate the truth, but miss it slightly. These "approximate" answers are typical.

The disorder is more common among males and has been seen in prisoners or people facing severe prison sentences or other disagreeable situations. There may be only one or two brief episodes or it may be chronic, but there often is a history of many prior hospitalizations and lifelong underachievement and instability.

This diagnosis is not made easily and must be differentiated from true psychosis and organic brain disorder. Testing by an expert psychologist may be of help.

Diagnostic Criteria for Factitious Disorder with Psychological Symptoms

A. The production of psychological symptoms which apparently are under voluntary control.
B. The symptoms are not explained by any other mental disorder even though superimposed on a severe personality disorder.
C. The individual's goal apparently is to assume to role of the patient and is not otherwise understandable.

FACTITIOUS DISORDER WITH PHYSICAL SYMPTOMS

This condition previously was called Munchausen's syndrome and is the most prevalent of the Factitious Disorders. The outstanding characteristic is the presentation of physical symptoms that are not real or are manufactured by the patient. The individual is able to present the symptoms so expertly and in such detail as to have obtained multiple hospitalizations, and many have had repeated diagnostic and surgical procedures. Some spend their entire lives being admitted to and staying in hospital, and every possible symptom and every know organ has been involved. Most hospital emergency rooms have pictures of and information on these individuals so that the personnel can be on the alert for them.

They present their histories with great dramatic flair and tend to arrive at emergency rooms at night when the less experienced people are on call. When extensive workups of their initial complaints fail to find any pathology, they usually invent other factitious symptoms and/or become very demanding, uncooperative, even threatening patients. They will discharge themselves against medical advice if bluntly confronted with the truth, but usually they go almost directly to some other hospital in another area.

The onset commonly is in early adult life, and these people ordinarily have few family ties, no steady employment, and few lasting relationships. Although the cause is unknown, it is not unusual to find the history of extensive medical treatment and hospitalization in childhood or adolescence with a tremendous grudge against the medical profession, yet a great need to be dependent upon doctors and nurses. These patients will undergo great pain and hardship to achieve their goal of medical treatment and hospitalization. The condition probably is far more common than it is recognized.

These people resemble those with Antisocial Personality Disorder to be discussed later, but the courses differ in that the Factitious Disorder has a later onset and the action has no goal other than to be hospitalized and to receive medical manipulations. The antisocial person works for more tangible, material goals.

Case Example

One man had obtained 57 known admissions to hospitals in the Midwest with the complaint of urinary bleeding. He had undergone innumerable cystoscopic examinations, bladder x-rays, and other diagnostic procedures. He produced his hematuria by inserting a wire with a small hook on it through the urethra, thereby producing lacerations of the bladder. When confronted with the truth in a V.A. hospital, even though it was done with kindness and understanding, he immediately left the hospital threatening to sue for malpractice. He next surfaced in a hospital over 300 miles away with the same complaint.

Diagnostic Criteria for Factitious Disorder with Physical Symptoms

A. Plausible presentation of physical symptoms that apparently are under the patient's voluntary control to such a degree that there are multiple hospitalizations.

B. The goal is to assume the role of a patient and is not otherwise understandable in the light of known circumstances.

TREATMENT

Successful treatment of Factitious Disorder with physical symptoms is rare because the patients are not motivated to change their behavior. In Factitious Disorder with Psychological Symptoms, the course may be brief and the symptoms may clear spontaneously once the stressful situation is over, but that is not true of the condition associated with physical symptoms. The patients in this group have been called "peregrinating" patients because they move from place to place and do not stay in one spot long enough to receive definitive psychiatric treatment. They produce anger, resentment, and eventual rejection in the medical profession–probably an unfair, although human, response.

Those with psychological symptoms should have a good evaluation and the offer of psychotherapy to help them mature enough to face reality. There are no specific medications and the patients tend to react badly to any and all drugs.

BIBLIOGRAPHY

Cramer, B., Gershberg, M., and Stern, M.: Munchausen syndrome. *Arch. Gen. Psychiatry, 24:*573, 1971.

Goldin, J., and MacDonald, J.: The ganser state. *J. Ment. Sci., 101:*267, 1955.

Spiro, H.: Chronic factitious illness: munchausen syndrome. *Arch. Gen. Psychiatry, 18:*569, 1968.

Whitlock, F.: The ganser syndrome. *Br. J. Psychiatry, 113:*19, 1967.

XVI

Disorders of Impulse Control

This group of interesting and sometimes serious conditions is characterized by three factors:

1. Failure to resist an impulse, drive, or temptation to perform some act that is harmful to the individual or others. The act may or may not be premeditated or planned and may or may not be consciously resisted.
2. An increasing sense of tension before beginning the act.
3. The experience of either pleasure, gratification, or relaxation at the time of committing the act. There may be genuine regret, self-reproach and guilt soon after the act, but not during the course of it.

Most of these disorders have a legal component primary or secondary to the act. Pyromania and Kleptomania are illegal acts, but Pathological Gambling, even where gambling is permitted, usually leads to legal problems secondary to losses or attempts to make good on losses. All impulse disorders produce some degree of chaos and misery in the family members.

DIAGNOSTIC CATEGORIES

Pathological Gambling

This is a chronic and progressive failure to resist the impulse to gamble even when the gambling behavior compromises, disrupts, or damages the person, family, or vocational pursuits. Gambling is a preoccupation which may become an irresistible obsession during periods of stress. All the possible complications of losses by gambling usually have occurred by the time these people are diagnosed. Many other antisocial behaviors may occur secondary to the need to pay off gambling debts, but the criminal behavior typically is nonviolent and the patient sincerely means to return or to pay back the money at that time. Many of these people become extremely uncomfortable if they win for a period of time, but may relax and feel normal after a loss that would make another person despondent.

Case Example

One victim of this disorder, a veteran of World War II and Korea, became severely depressed and was hospitalized on a V.A. psychiatric ward after having won over $100,000 in a marathon poker game. He did not recover from the depression in spite of intensive treatment for several weeks. He left the hospital against medical advice and took his large sum of cash with him. He came back by the psychiatric ward several days later to tell his doctor that he had lost all his money, but that he was feeling well. He also told that he had been depressed several times in the past when he had won large sums of money.

There may be many predisposing factors such as hyperexposure to gambling in childhood and adolescence or living in a family which set a high value on material and financial symbols, but the true cause is unknown. It is much more common among males than females, and the families of origin have a higher than average incidence of alcoholism and other forms of impulsive behavior.

Diagnostic Criteria for Pathological Gambling

A. The individual is chronically and progressively unable to resist the impulse to gamble.

B. Gambling compromises, disrupts, or damages family, personal, and vocational pursuits as indicated by at least two of the following:

 1. Arrest for forgery, fraud, embezzlement, or other illegal attempts to obtain money for gambling

2. Defaults on debts and other responsibilities
3. Family disruption
4. Borrowing of money from illegal sources
5. Inability to account for loss of money or to produce evidence of winning, if this is claimed
6. Loss of work due to absenteeism in order to pursue gambling activity
7. Necessity for another person to provide money to relieve a desperate financial sitatuion

C. The condition is not due to Antisocial Personality Disorder or to other mental disease.

Kleptomania

This is the recurrent failure to resist the impulse to steal objects which are not for immediate use or for their monetary value. The objects may be given away, returned surreptitiously, or stored and, almost invariably, the individual could have obtained the object more easily by paying for it or asking for it. These people usually perform the act under tension, but they confess a feeling of intense gratification during the act. Frequently the theft is made in such a way that detection is almost certain, and true Kleptomania always is a solitary act. Shoplifting or any form of theft done in cooperation with another person is not Kleptomania.

Many of these people show signs of depression and guilt over the knowledge of what they have done, but others may act as if the whole thing were a joke and unimportant. The condition waxes and wanes, but tends to begin in early childhood or adolescence. The major complications are the social and legal difficulties which the stealing produces and the family upsets secondary to it.

Case Example

A minister's teen-aged daughter was obsessed with stealing small shiny objects and pens of all types. She was a plain, overweight, and unattractive girl with two handsome older siblings who were the pride of the family. She felt unloved and unwanted and often had daydreamed that she had been adopted. She invariably left the stolen objects where a parent was certain to find them. Kleptomania had many meanings to her, but the superficial one was the attention it attracted to her. She also found it a way to embarrass and shame her over-righteous father, especially when she was caught stealing in a shop which was owned by a member of her father's congregation.

Diagnostic Criteria for Kleptomania

A. Recurrent failure to resist impulses to steal objects that are not for immediate use or monetary value.
B. Increasing sense of tension before the act.
C. Pleasure or release of tension at the time of committing the theft.
D. Stealing without long-term planning and without assistance from others.
E. Not due to an Antisocial Personality Disorder or a mental illness.

Pyromania

This much more serious condition is the recurrent failure to resist impulses to set fires and an intense fascination with watching them burn. There is the usual buildup of anxiety before the act, and the usual release of tension and feeling of euphoria once the fire is underway.

Many of these people are chronic "firewatchers" and frequently set off false alarms just to see the firefighting apparatus in action. Unfortunately, they are overrepresented among people who work or have worked in or about fire departments. They tend to be people with other personality disorders including alcoholism, low I.Q., and a poor set of personal standards and values. The major consequences are legal. The pyromaniac's past history may reveal an overaverage childhood fascination with fire, matches, and flames, but by no means does every child who plays with matches become a pyromaniac.

Diagnostic Criteria for Pyromania

A. Recurrent failure to resist impulses to set fires.

B. Increasing sense of tension before setting the fire.
C. The experience of pleasure, gratification, or relaxation at the time of setting the fire.
D. Lack of motivation, other than psychological, for setting the fire.
E. Not due to Organic Mental Disorder, Schizophrenia, or other Conduct or Personality Disorder.

Intermittent Explosive Disorder

The essential features are several separate episodes of loss of control of aggressive impulses that have resulted in serious assault or destruction. The degree of aggression expressed during an episode is out of proportion to any precipitating stress. The people may describe these episodes as "spells." These spells may come on rapidly and dissipate just as quickly. Regret, guilt, and self-reproach may follow each episode, and the patient truly may wish to be helped. Episodes may be signalled by some change in sensory feelings or behavior, but these usually cannot be observed by associates. Friends and relatives describe these people as having a "bad temper."

The condition must be carefully differentiated from an Organic Brain Disorder, especially one that may be due to a form of epilepsy arising from areas in the temporal lobes of the brain. A careful psychiatric and neurological examination must be done before this diagnosis is made. Past history may include head trauma and/or infections from which there was an apparent complete recovery.

Case Example

A 30-year-old man came for psychiatric consultation after he had broken his wife's nose when she had overcooked his breakfast eggs! He gave a history of violent outbursts at slight provocation for about five years, but both he and his wife felt that the frequency of tantrums was increasing. He also told of spells of feeling "peculiar" in his head many times when he did not explode. A year before the first know violent episode the man had severe Herpes Zoster on the chest. He had been quite ill and took many months for complete recovery.

An electroencephalogram showed slow waves and spikes coming from the right temporal lobe. Anticonvulsant drugs reduced his episodes by 90%, although an occasional outburst was reported. This case exemplifies the need for suspicion of organic lesions when the diagnosis of Intermittent Explosive Disorder is suspected.

Diagnostic Criteria for Intermittent Explosive Disorder

A. Several discrete episodes of loss of control of aggressive impulses resulting in serious assault or destruction of property.
B. Behavior that is grossly out of proportion to any precipitating psychosocial stressor.
C. Absence of signs of generalized impulsivity or aggressiveness between episodes.
D. Not due to Schizophrenia, Antisocial Personality Disorder, or Conduct Disorder.

Isolated Explosive Disorder

This refers to one discrete episode of failure to resist an impulse that led to a single, violent, externally directed act with a catastrophic impact on others. Careful consideration must be given for some more deep-seated pathologies such as Paranoid Type Schizophrenia or brain dysfunction due to an organic lesion.

Case Example

The young man who sat in a tower on a Texas campus and shot more than 20 people had no previous history suggesting such a disorder. He had been an excellent student, a good marine, and a devoted family member. There was no observable precipitating cause, and his past history gave no hint that he was liable to be dangerous. An autopsy showed a small brain tumor, but it was in an area that made it doubtful that it caused the explosive behavior.

Diagnostic Criteria for Isolated Explosive Disorder

A. A single discrete episode in which failure to resist an impulse led to a single violent act which had a catastrophic effect. The degree of aggressivity during the episode was grossly out of proportion to any precipitating stress.

B. The episodes were not preceded by signs of generalized impulsivity or aggressiveness.
C. Not due to any other mental or emotional illness.

TREATMENT

All Impulse Disorder victims must have a thorough examination to rule out organic brain pathology. Treatment primarily is some form of psychotherapy or behavioral modification. Group therapy and self-help groups have been successful, especially with Pathological Gambling. Medications are of little value. The legal consequences of these conditions may complicate the situation and always must be considered in a treatment program.

Kleptomania cannot be properly treated without involving the family of the young person.

BIBLIOGRAPHY

Bolen, W., and Boyd, W.: Gambling and the gambler. *Arch. Gen. Psychiatry, 18:*617, 1968.

Frosch, W.: The relation between acting out and disorders of impulse control. *Psychiatry, 40:*295, 1977.

Harbin, H.: Episodic dyscontrol and family dynamics. *Am. J. Psychiatry, 134:*1113, 1977.

Keutzer, C.: Kleptomania: a direct approach to treatment. *Br. J. Med. Psychology, 45:*159, 1972.

Mavromatis, M., and Lion, J.: A primer on pyromania. *Dis. Ner. Sys., 38:*954, 1977.

XVII

Adjustment Disorders

This diagnosis requires a maladaptive reaction to an identifiable psychosocial stressor within no more than three months after the stressful event. There must be impairment in social or occupational functioning or symptoms that obviously are in excess of an expected reaction to the stress. A mother who temporarily became nonfunctional following the accidental death of her child would not be diagnosed as having an Adjustment Disorder since that is an expected reaction appropriate to the stress.

Most Adjustment Disorders will remit eventually or, if the stress is unrelenting, a new level of adaptation will be achieved. The stressors may be single, as in an accident or divorce, or multiple, such as a series of family or business difficulties. Individuals or even whole communities can be affected, as was true of a small Kentucky town when a broken dam flooded and destroyed most of the village and its people. Later research showed that almost the entire group of survivors went through a severe Adjustment Disorder.

It is important to be able to judge the individual in relation to the stress. Many people are more vulnerable to particular types of stresses depending upon innate coping abilities, the private meaning of the stressor, and upon environmental factors. (See Chapter 2 on Stress.) The key factor in the diagnosis must be the maladaptive response and the element of time. Individuals with preexisting Personality Disorders or with some form of brain disease may be much more vulnerable to stress as are those people with deficiencies in social supports.

ADJUSTMENT DISORDER

Diagnostic Criteria

A. A maladaptive reaction to an identifiable psychosocial stressor within three months of the onset of the stress.
B. The maladaptive nature of the reaction is indicated by either of the following:
   1. Impairment in social or occupational functioning
   2. Symptoms that are in excess of a normal and expected reaction
C. The disturbance is not merely one instance of a pattern of overreaction to stress or an exacerbation of some other mental disorder.
D. It is assumed that the disturbance will remit in a period of time or, if the stress persists, that a new level of adaptation will be achieved.

SUB-TYPES OF ADJUSTMENT DISORDER

Adjustment Disorder with Depressed Mood

This category means that the predominant manifestation involves symptoms of depressed mood, tearfulness, and feelings of hopelessness, but the condition must be differentiated from true depression and uncomplicated grief. A major factor in grief is that it is not a maladaptive response when it is appropriate to a realistic loss.

Case Example

Jane was seen with the story that she had been crying periodically for several days, had been unable to do her work as a secretary properly, and felt that life was not worth living. She had no other signs of depression such as sleep disturbance or loss of appetite. The symptoms had begun the week after her financé of several months had told her that he wanted to continue their relationship, but not at the previous level. He felt that they should date other people and see less of each other for a few months, then reassess their engagement. There were some elements of both depression and grief in Jane's reaction, but the severity of her symptoms did not warrant a diagnosis of depression and a grief response would have been inappropriate.

Adjustment Disorder with Anxious Mood

The major symptoms involve nervousness, worry, chronic tenseness, and hyperexcitability: the usual symptoms of anxiety.

Adjustment Disorder with Mixed Emotional Features

Occasionally one sees the symptoms of anxiety and depression intermingled in various combinations so that neither dominates the picture.

Adjustment Disorder with Disturbance of Conduct

There may be no emotional signs and symptoms, but family and friends may note a marked change in previous behavior. This may include truancy, vandalism, fighting, drug abuse, and other forms of illegal activity or breaking of social norms. The involved person may be unaware of any change in feeling.

Adjustment Disorder with Mixed Disturbances of Emotions and Conduct

This refers to the conduct disturbances listed above combined with the symptoms of depression and/or anxiety.

Adjustment Disorder with Work (or Academic) Inhibition

There may be no physical or emotional signs, but the individual may demonstrate, at work or at school, a marked decline in the usual level of performance. One should always suspect some other form of anxiety or depression before making this diagnosis.

Adjustment Disorder with Withdrawal

The major sign is a complete withdrawal from usual social activities.

Case Example

A 50-year-old woman who ran a large, successful family business became depressed, tearful, and nonfunctional within a week of learning that her previously trusted son had embezzled money which had left the business on the verge of bankruptcy. She was unable to cooperate with the authorities for approximately three weeks and cancelled all social engagements, but gradually regained her original level of function after four sessions of psychotherapy.

TREATMENT

Medications

Occasional short-term use of antianxiety drugs or sedatives is both helpful and humane. That is especially true in the conditions with anxious mood or in the one with mixed disturbances of emotions and conduct. Short-term means from 10 to 14 days in the lowest effective dose.

Psychotherapy

A form of supportive psychotherapy which may be given by professionals or by pastors, family, and friends usually is helpful. This allows the individual to express the basic feelings openly, to identify the stressor as fully as possible, and to explore alternative methods of adjustment to the changed situation.

One must be alert to the possibility of an Adjustment Disorder progressing into a more serious condition in predisposed people. It is possible for an Adjustment Disorder with Depressed Mood to slip into a Major Depressive Disorder and require more definitive treatment. The risk is particularly great if there is a past history of depression in the patient or the patient's family.

BIBLIOGRAPHY

Furst, S.: *Psychic Trauma.* New York, Basic Books, 1967.

Langsley, D., and Kaplan, D.: *The Treatment of Families in Crisis.* New York, Grune & Stratton, 1968.

Pollock, G.: Anniversary reactions, trauma and mourning. *Psychoanalytic Quarterly, 39:*347, 1970.

Selye, H.: *The Stress of Life.* New York, McGraw-Hill, 1978.

XVIII

Personality Disorders

The human personality is the sum total of every stimulus that has impinged upon that individual since conception. The effects of those stimuli will depend much on the genetic background, the social and cultural context, and many of those factors discussed under the chapter on Functional Illness. The final personality is a collection of traits which are enduring patterns of perceiving, relating to, and thinking about oneself and the environment. A Personality Disorder arises only when those traits are inflexible and maladaptive and cause either significant impairment in social or occupational functioning or distress to the individual. Personality Disorders generally are identifiable by adolescence or very early adulthood and continue relatively unchanged throughout life. The individual with a Personality Disorder tends to be unaware of it (denial) and usually becomes uncomfortable only because of the reaction of the environment to the personality, not because of the symptoms of the Personality Disorder *per se*.

Some form of a depression or anxiety is common in people with Personality Disorders. These feelings tend to occur when the Personality Disorder produces difficulty with social and/or occupational endeavors. A man with a Paranoid Personality may feel perfectly justified in all of his feelings and thoughts, but may become anxious and depressed when he loses a job because of his constant suspicions and distrustfulness.

SPECIFIC PERSONALITY DISORDERS

There is much overlap and intermingling of the symptomatology of the Personality Disorders, but a specific diagnosis is made when a given set of signs and symptoms produce a relatively fixed pattern of behavior. An exact diagnosis requires a very thorough study of the individual, including detailed information as to how family, friends, and associates see that person.

Paranoid Personality Disorder

The outstanding picture is a pervasive and unwarranted suspiciousness and mistrust of people, hypersensitivity, and a constant tendency to blame others or the environment for all mishaps.

Distrust and suspicion may be quite justified and adaptive in many difficult life situations. If the attitudes are not justified, a mature individual will abandon them when given convincing evidence to the contrary, but a Paranoid Personality Disorder not only ignores evidence of reality when it conflicts with a belief, but becomes very suspicious of those who present the evidence. They feel that people either are for or against them; rarely is there a middle ground. They are guarded, devious,and almost always extremely jealous. They are constantly on the lookout for hidden motives and special meanings, and act as if "the best defense is a good offense." Usually, they lack humor and tend to avoid soft, emotional feelings. They see emotionality and empathy as weaknesses or as ploys to get close to them so as to hurt them.

The person with a Paranoid Personality Disorder frequently is ambitious and capable and may be quite successful because of stubbornness and a tendency to persevere. They work best alone and are poor group workers who may be much more comfortable with objects than with people. They respect and fear power and authority, but at the same time are envious and jealous of it and strive to achieve it. They tend to think concretely and to have little time for nuances and subtleties.

The cause of the disorder is unknown, but there seems to be a familial pattern, some of which may be genetic and some of which may be learned from parents who have taught the child that the world is dangerous and that every man is out for himself.

Diagnostic Criteria for Paranoid Personality Disorder

A. Pervasive, unwarranted suspiciousness and mistrust of people as indicated by at least three of the following:
   1. Expectation of trickery or harm
   2. Hypervigilance
   3. Guardedness or secretiveness
   4. Avoidance of accepting blame
   5. Questioning the loyalty of others
   6. Intense, narrowly-focused searching for confirmation of personal bias with loss of appreciation of the total picture
   7. Overconcern with hidden motives and special meanings
   8. Jealousy
B. Hypersensitivity as indicated by at least two of the following:
   1. Tendency to be easily slighted and quick to take offense
   2. Exaggeration of difficulties
   3. Readiness to counterattack when any threat is perceived
   4. The inability to relax
C. Restricted affectivity as indicated by at least two of the following:
   1. Appearance of being cold and unemotional
   2. Pride in their objective, rational, and unemotional attitudes
   3. Lack of a true sense of humor
   4. Absence of passive, soft, and sentimental feelings

Schizoid Personality Disorder

The necessary feature is a defect in the capacity to form social relationships as manifested by the absence of close feelings for others and indifference to praise, criticism, and the welfare of others. There will be no other eccentricities of speech, behavior, or thought. These individuals show no desire for social involvement and prefer to be "loners" and to pursue solitary, withdrawn interests and hobbies. Others see them as cold, aloof, humorless, and dull. They usually express neither great aggressivity or emotional involvement and are given to excessive day-dreaming.

These individuals may be capable of high level functioning in situations where they can work alone without concern for social considerations. The condition often is obvious by mid-adolescence and, since these people are not uncomfortable with their situation, it often is chronic.

Case Example

A 19-year-old boy was brought for consultation by parents who wanted him to be popular and active like his older brother. He had no close friends, never had dated, and occupied himself solely with studies and his hobby of electronics. A school testing program had rated his I.Q. at 130.

The young man cooperated in the interview by answering all questions as simply as possible, but he volunteered nothing and showed no sign of emotion one way or the other. He stated calmly, but convincingly, that he had no interest in being a "social butterfly," and while he expressed regret at his parents' discomfort with him, he intended to continue as he was.

Diagnostic Criteria for Schizoid Personality Disorder

A. Emotional coldness and aloofness and absence of warm, tender feelings for others.
B. Indifference to praise or criticism and to the feelings of others.
C. Close friendships with no more than one or two persons.
D. No eccentricities of speech, behavior, or thought characteristic of Schizotypal Personality Disorders.
E. Not due to a psychotic disorder.

Schizotypal Personality Disorder

This condition is characterized by various eccentricities of thought, perception, speech, and behavior which are not severe enough to meet the criteria for Schizophrenia. No single feature is invariably present, but one sees magical thinking, bizarre fantasies, ideas of reference and, perhaps, some paranoid feeling. The eccentricities usually interfere with social functioning so that other people tend to avoid them. Under stress there may be periods that almost resemble Schizophrenia in that there may be feelings of depersonalization and recurrent illusions (not delusions). These individuals are prone to peculiar convictions such as fanaticism, belief in fringe religious sects, and adherence to questionable political and ethical groups or codes.

The incidence of Schizophrenia is above the average among family members of individuals with Schizotypal Personality Disorder, and some psychiatrists feel that it represents a borderline or marginal type of Schizophrenia which may become blatant under stress.

Case Example

A college coed's parents told of their daughter's eccentricities and wanted to know what they should do. They described her as "strange," and told of her preoccupation with witchcraft since early adolescence. She had few associates except those she met at the many fringe organizations she attended. She dressed in a bizarre fashion and appeared immune to the stares and jibes of her classmates. She became emotional when her odd beliefs were challenged, but usually acted as if others' opinions did not matter to her.

The girl refused to have a psychiatric consultation, and shortly after her parents had spoken to her of it, she became a full-time member of an obscure religious cult.

Diagnostic Criteria for Schizotypal Personality Disorder

A. At least four of the following:
   1. Magical thinking such as superstitiousness, clairvoyance, telepathy, belief in extrasensory perception, bizarre fantasies, and fanatic attachments.
   2. Ideas of reference
   3. Social isolation
   4. Recurrent illusions such as sensing the presence of a force or person not actually there, depersonalization, or derealization not associated with panic attacks

5. Odd speech, but without loosening of associations or incoherence
6. Inadequate ability to relate well to others due to constricted or inappropriate affect (feelings)
7. Suspiciousness or paranoid ideation
8. Undue anxiety or hypersensitivity to real or imagined criticism in social situations

Histrionic Personality Disorder

The essential characteristic is a Personality Disorder in which there are overly dramatic, reactive, and intensely expressed behavior and characteristic disturbances in interpersonal relationships. These people are prone to exaggeration, "hamming it up," and always attempt to draw attention to themselves. They are prone to emotional outbursts which are inappropriate to the stimulus and which occur only in the presence of others. These individuals often are very charming and appealing when things go well for them, but they are shallow and lack the ability to form close relationships unless they expect to profit from them. Suicidal gestures, eccentric manipulations, and an uncanny ability to persuade other people to do things for them are seen. They tend to control the opposite sex by seduction, but their sexual relationships often are shallow and unsatisfactory.

These people show little interest in achievement except as it brings them personal attention. Their intense self-involvement makes them susceptible to depressions when frustrated or ignored. They are very suggestible and sensitive, and frequent complaints of physical and/or mental symptoms lead to much doctor shopping. Hysterical episodes take them to emergency rooms at an above average rate.

Case Example

Ms. N. was brought to the emergency room by an ambulance after a "choking" episode in a restaurant. Her spell of choking, shortness of breath, rapid heart rate and tingling of hands and feet came on when her boyfriend told her that he was moving to another state without her.

She had a lifelong history of nervous spells when rejected, neglected, or frustrated. She was a beautiful woman known as a "clothes horse" by her friends. Although almost 40 years old, she dressed and looked as much as possible like a late adolescent. She had been married and divorced three times and had had many love affairs. Later, in psychotherapy, she admitted that sex was something she could take or leave, but that it was useful for controlling men.

Diagnostic Criteria for Histrionic Personality Disorder

A. Behavior that is overly dramatic, reactive and intensely expressed as manifested by at least three of the following:
  1. Self-dramatization and exaggerated expressions of emotions
  2. Incessant drawing of attention to self
  3. Craving for activity and excitement
  4. Overreaction to minor events
  5. Irrational, angry outbursts, or tantrums

B. Characteristic disturbance in interpersonal relationships as manifested by at least two of the following:
  1. Perceived by others as shallow and lacking in genuineness, even if superficially warm and charming
  2. Egocentric, self-indulgent and inconsiderate
  3. Vain and demanding
  4. Dependent, helpless, constantly seeking reassurance
  5. Prone to manipulative suicide threats, gestures, or attempts

Narcissistic Personality Disorder

The name of this condition describes it perfectly: exaggerated self-love. These people have a grandiose sense of uniqueness and a preoccupation with what they see as unlimited successes and abilities. They need constant attention and admiration and, if they do not receive it, can become very unlikable and peevish. Many have grandiose expectations of themselves which may lead to a sense of failure if perfection is not achieved quickly.

The narcissistic person may achieve success in a given field, but it never gives self-satisfaction since the admiration and rewards will not equal the expectations. The outward show of extreme self-love may appear fragile when there is a disappointment or a defeat and these people decompensate into rage, humiliation, and shame out of keeping with reality.

The person with a Narcissistic Personality Disorder is not well-liked because of the complete self-centeredness and lack of empathy. Their expectations that others will always do for them without thought of payment or thanks leads to unrewarding relationships. If they attempt to make friends, they usually do so for some personal gain. They are incapable of ordinary love and affection for others.

Case Example

A 25-year-old graduate student was seen in consultation at the urging of his immediate supervisor who thought that he was a disruptive force in the program. The student approached the interview with a haughty, disdainful air and called the psychiatrist by his first name. He readily admitted that he had no use for his colleagues whom he termed "2nd raters and also-rans." He spoke of his many love affairs, but later admitted that most were one-night stands since the women never were his social equals. He boasted of his superior education at an Ivy League school. He told of grandiose plans for his research, hinting at a possible Nobel Prize.

It was learned months later that his research project never was completed.

Diagnostic Criteria for Narcissistic Personality Disorder

A. Grandiose sense of self-importance or uniqueness with exaggeration of achievements and talents.
B. Preoccupations with fantasies of unlimited success, power, or any other ideal.
C. Exhibitionism
D. Indifference or feeling of rage, inferiority, and humiliation in response to criticism or to lack of attention from others.

E. At least two of the following characteristic disturbances in interpersonal relationships:
   1. Entitlement (The world should reward me!)
   2. Interpersonal exploitativeness
   3. Relationships that characteristically alternate between the extremes of overidealization and devaluation
   4. Lack of empathy

Antisocial Personality Disorder

This may be the most important of the Personality Disorders in view of the tragedy, disharmony, and economic loss the condition can produce in society and in families. It is characterized by a history of continuous and chronic antisocial behavior in which the rights of others are violated, by onset before age 15 with persistence into adult life, and by failure to sustain the expected social performances. It is a condition in which lying, stealing, fighting, truancy, and resistance to authority are typical childhood signs which tend to progress in adolescence to acting-out of all forms including drugs, alcohol, and sex.

Antisocial Personality is an example of a Superego deficiency. A deficient or faulty Superego means that the individual has little if any guilt and anxiety such as most people feel when acting contrary to an internalized set of standards and values. These are self-centered people who feel that "it is coming to them" and that they are justified in whatever means it takes to protect themselves or get what they want. A close and responsible relationship with any other person is rare. They see other people and things only in terms of profit to themselves. The fact that they do not feel normal guilt or anxiety means that these people rarely voluntarily seek assistance.

These are the con-men, the flimflams, the Elmer Gantries of the world. The condition is much more common in males than females, and there is a strong suggestion that there is an inherited factor. This genetic component and an early environment which prevents development of a workable set of values and standards by identification with a responsible parent figure are strong etiological factors.

Case Example

J.D. made a half-hearted suicide attempt while in jail for stealing a credit card and spending thousands of dollars with it. He begged for help and was released on the agreement that he would enter psychotherapy.

His history was one of trouble with authorities since the sixth grade. He had made it through high school primarily because his parents were influential people in the community. In the seven years since high school graduation, he had been enrolled in three colleges and had held many jobs, but none for over two months at a time.

J.D. was a heavy user of street drugs and alcohol. He had been in two drug treatment programs, but completed neither. He always quit the programs when the legal pressure was removed.

He remained in psychotherapy for two months after the suicide attempt, just long enough to get the charges dropped.

Diagnostic Criteria for Antisocial Personality Disorder

A. The current age at least 18

B. Onset before age 15 as indicated by a history of three or more of the following:

1. Truancy
2. Expulsion or suspension from school or misbehavior
3. Delinquency
4. Running away from home overnight at least twice
5. Persistent lying
6. Repeated sexual intercourse in a casual relationship
7. Repeated drunkenness or substance abuse
8. Thefts
9. Vandalism
10. School grades markedly below expectations and abilities
11. Chronic violators of rules at home, school, or other social agencies
12. Initiation of fights

C. At least four of the following manifestations of the disorder since age 18:
   1. Inability to sustain consistent work or school behavior
   2. Lack of ability to function as a responsible parent
   3. Failure to accept social norms with respect to lawful behavior
   4. Inability to maintain enduring attachments to a sexual partner as indicated by divorces and/or separations
   5. Irritability and aggressiveness as indicated by repeated physical fights and assaults
   6. Failure to honor financial obligations
   7. Failure to plan ahead and/or impulsivity
   8. Disregard for the truth
   9. Recklessness in any and all other behavior

D. A pattern of continuous antisocial behavior in which the rights of others are violated with no intervening "normal" periods for at least five years.

Borderline Personality Disorder

Older texts will use the title "borderline" to refer to individuals who are on the border between being "normal" and psychotic, usually schizophrenic. The modern use of the term is characterized by instability in a variety of areas including interpersonal behavior, mood, and self-image. Interpersonal relations are fluid and marked with shifts of attitude over time, impulsive and unpredictable behavior, and potentially self-damaging behavior. The mood shifts rapidly and inappropriately from one extreme to the other and these people complain constantly of boredom and feelings of emptiness.

There may be an admixture of many of the features discussed under Schizotypal, Histrionic, Narcissistic, and Antisocial Personality Disorders. A brief psychotic episode under stress is not unusual.

The disorder is most commonly diagnosed in women, and some form of depression is the most frequent reason for asking for psychiatric help.

Case Example

Ms. J. was admitted to the psychiatric service after superficially cutting both wrists following a quarrel with her husband which ended with him moving out of their house for the fourth time in three years of marriage. She was petulant and demanding as soon as she was admitted, but was coy and seductive with the male psychiatrist assigned to her.

Ms. J. had a history of two previous suicidal gestures, both following perceived rejections by busy friends. She told of chronic boredom unless life was a series of parties and exciting events. She was a very attractive female, but felt that she was an "ugly duckling" from whom men wanted only one thing–sex. She continued in psychotherapy after leaving the hospital, but discontinued it when she and her husband were reconciled.

Diagnostic Criteria for Borderline Personality Disorder

A. At least five of the following are required:
   1. Impulsivity or unpredictability in at least two areas that are potentially self-damaging
   2. A pattern of unstable and intense interpersonal relationships
   3. Inappropriate, intense anger or lack of control of anger
   4. Identity disturbance manifested by uncertainty about several issues relating to self-image, gender identity, long-term goals or career choices, friendship patterns, values, and/or loyalties.
   5. Affective instability with mood shifts of short duration
   6. Intolerance of being alone
   7. Physically self-damaging acts and gestures
   8. Chronic feelings of emptiness or boredom

B. The patient must be over 18 years of age.

Avoidant Personality Disorder

You will note that the name of the disorder describes it succinctly. The outstanding feature of this disorder is hypersensitivity to potential rejection, humiliation, or shame so that the individual avoids entering into relationships without unusually strong guarantees of blanket acceptance. These individuals may be devastated by the slightest hint of disapproval so that an already low self-esteem becomes no self-esteem. The condition differs from Schizoid Personality Disorder in that the Avoidant Personality victim yearns for affection and acceptance and is distressed by the lack of ability to "belong." The Schizoid person does not want to belong.

This condition apparently is common in adolescence and young adulthood, and the major affect caused by it is depression. It is the depression that brings the patient to medical attention. The condition may coexist with a simple phobia.

Case Example

A 21-year-old college senior went to the Student Health Clinic with complaints of inability to concentrate resulting in falling grades, insomnia, loss of appetite, and a general feeling that life was not worth living. A thorough history from the student plus information from her family revealed a typical Avoidant Personality Disorder obvious since puberty. She came from a large, close family unit in which no one was aware of the severity of her personality problems, although they encouraged her constantly to be more socially active. The longer she was in college away from the family, the more distressed she became by her lack of ability to relate to others. She sought treatment not for the Personality Disorder, but for the depressive symptoms which it had produced.

Diagnostic Criteria for Avoidant Personality Disorder

A. Hypersensitivity to rejection.
B. Unwillingness to enter into relationships without a guarantee of uncritical acceptance.
C. Social withdrawal.
D. Desire for affection and acceptance.
E. Low self-esteem.

Dependent Personality Disorder

This individual passively allows others to assume responsibility for major areas of existence because of a lack of self-confidence and an inability to function independently. Any sacrifice or act may be done to avoid the possibility of having to be self-reliant. Persons with this disorder are unwilling to make demands on others for fear of jeopardizing the relationship, and this may progress to taking tremendous abuse and to being victimized. Decision-making is avoided until someone tells the Dependent Personality what to do.

These people may function well in a relationship with someone who wishes to tolerate this dependency and be a nurturing boss, but anxiety and depression are common when the relationship terminates. The condition is more common in females.

Case Example

Miss A. was seen with a prolonged Adjustment Disorder after the death of her father with whom she had lived all her 46 years. Her mother had died when she was 16 and, except for a few dates in her early 20s, she had devoted her life to keeping her father's house. Her sole outside activity was church attendance every Sunday. She had no ideas of finance, not even how to write a check to pay bills. Other than keeping his clothing and shopping for groceries, she had been totally dependent on her father, both financially and emotionally. She had several close friends in the community, and all the neighborhood children knew her as a kind, generous lady always good for some cake or cookies.

Miss A. transferred her dependence to the psychotherapist, but a year later she was working as a teacher's aid, had bought an automobile, and was considering a tour to Europe on the money left by her father.

Diagnostic Criteria for Dependent Personality Disorder

A. Passively allows others to assume responsibility for major areas of existence.
B. Subordinates own needs to those of others on whom a dependent relationship is possible in order to avoid self-reliance.
C. Lacks self-confidence.

Compulsive Personality Disorder

Whereas it was said that the Antisocial Personality has a defective Superego, the Compulsive Personality Disorder has one that is too strong, inflexible, and punitive. These are perfectionists with a restricted ability to express warm and tender emotions, insistence that others submit to their way of doing things, excessive devotion to work and to productivity to the exclusion of pleasure, and chronic indecisiveness. They tend to be stingy with both emotions and material goods and preoccupied with rules, efficiency, trivia, forms, and procedures. They are "list makers" and "doubting Thomases" who may spend more time thinking about and enumerating tasks than in doing them.

They work at pleasure, if they have any at all. It is as if their lives are controlled by guilt which must be atoned for by sacrifice and self-denial. Their major distresses come from their indecisiveness and from the distress they produce in others who must work with them and around them. No one pleases them completely, and they never please themselves sufficiently to be satisfied. They are excessively conscientious, moralistic, and very judgmental of self and others.

The disorder, an apparently common one, occurs most frequent in men. It appears to run in families, and the parents of the Compulsive Personality Disorder often have been people who were upwardly mobile, very concerned with production and with what others thought of them. They tended to reward the child with love and approval for high achievement, but to withhold love when the child failed to produce.

Case Example

B. was an assistant professor of mathematics at an Eastern university. He became depressed and nonfunctional when refused promotion and tenure. He was a 38-year-old bachelor who lived in an immaculate apartment which he cleaned completely every Sunday. His life was regimented by a notebook in which he listed every hour's activities weekly. He refused to deviate from the list, but almost never completed the things he was scheduled to do.

B. could agonize for a half-day over buying a shirt. He always doubted a decision as soon as he made it. He had closets of clothing which had never been worn since he was saving them for the future.

Students detested him since his lectures were filled with minute details and trivia which he expected them to memorize. He wrote and rewrote lectures many times, but always thought that he had left out something important.

Diagnostic Criteria for Compulsive Personality Disorder

At least four of the following are characteristic of the current and long-term functioning and cause either significant impairment in social or occupational functioning or subjective distress:

1. Restricted ability to express warm and tender emotions
2. Perfectionism that interferes with the ability to grasp the "whole picture," such as preoccupation with trivial details and lists
3. Insistence that others submit to their way of doing things and a lack of awareness of the feelings elicited by this behavior
4. Excessive devotion to work and productivity
5. Indecisiveness which culminates in delay, fear of mistakes, and ruminating about priorities

Passive-Aggressive Personality Disorder

The two parts of this compound name, "passive-aggressive," appear to be contradictory. The essential feature is a resistance to demands for adequate performance in both occupational and social functioning, but the resistance is expressed indirectly rather than directly. The name is based on the assumption that these individuals are passively expressing hidden aggression.

These people habitually resent and resist demands to maintain a given level of functioning. The resistance is expressed indirectly through procrastination, dawdling, stubbornness, "forgetfulness," and errors. Habitual lateness may infuriate employers, family, and colleagues, but may become a standing joke or be done in such a way that the culprit cannot be openly reprimanded. These people become adept at producing anger and resentment in others, but doing it in such a way that the victimized ones cannot retaliate without feeling guilty or ashamed.

The people with this disorder are not consciously aware of their anger and aggressivity. They are pessimistic about the future, but fail to realize that their own personalities produce this lack of optimism. They are aware of their resentment of authority, but not aware of its effect on their behavior. When confronted with their behavior, they act hurt and concerned, but they do not change.

Case Example

Dr. C. was an assistant professor of medicine. He exasperated the departmental chairman and the secretarial staff with his behavior. Records never were completed on time, reports were chronically late, but Dr. C. always promised to catch up immediately. This did not happen, or if it did, it was temporary.

Dr. C. was quiet, charming, and unassuming on the surface. His constant lateness always could be explained, and if fellow workers became irritated he acted as if he were the injured party. When his chairman explained the problem to him, C. was surprised that there was a problem, but changed his behavior immediately. It lasted two weeks.

Diagnostic Criteria for Passive-Aggressive Personality Disorder

A. Resistance to demands for adequate performance in both occupational and social functioning

B. Resistance expressed indirectly through at least two of the following:

   1. Procrastination
   2. Dawdling
   3. Stubborness
   4. Intentional inefficiency
   5. "Forgetfulness"

C. As a consequence of A and B, pervasive and long-standing social and occupational ineffectiveness.

D. Persistence of the behavior pattern even under circumstances in which more self-assertive and effective behavior is possible.

TREATMENT

People with Personality Disorders ordinarily do not volunteer for treatment because they rarely feel that they are ill or, if they do, they feel that it is someone else's fault. If they become patients, they ordinarily do so because of outside pressure from friends, family, or employers, or because of depression or anxiety secondary to society's reaction to their behavior.

Medications

Medications have little use in the treatment of Personality Disorders, but may be useful in the treatment of secondary symptoms such as anxiety and depression. Whether to use these medications will depend upon the severity of the symptomatology and on the knowledge that they are temporary and symptomatic treatments only.

Psychotherapy

Expert psychoanalytically oriented psychotherapy may be of value in many of the Personality Disorders when something occurs to motivate the patient for change. This motivation usually is secondary to the symptomatology or outside pressure. A therapist who can make a close relationship with one of these individuals must be patient, empathetic, and understanding over a long period of time. There is no magic formula or shortcut. The specific disorders may require different psychotherapeutic approaches. For example, an immediate show of empathy and closeness may be necessary in the Avoidant Personality Disorder, but contraindicated in a person with a Paranoid Personality Disorder. At least in the beginning, treatment with the Paranoid Personality Disorder should be kept on an intellectual plane and the degree of closeness left entirely up to the patient.

One of the Personality Disorders requires more specific information about treatment. The Antisocial Disorder, if of any severity, is very difficult to treat and may be impossible to treat outside a close environment. Treatment not only is unsuccessful, but there is a degree of danger that these individuals may increase their antisocial activities if they become anxious about themselves during the treatment process. Successful treatment usually requires complete control over the environment of the patient (milieu therapy) for prolonged periods of time. Results are questionable under the best of circumstances but, fortunately, the Antisocial Personality frequently "burns out" and changes for the better somewhere in the middle years of life. Old "sociopaths," the popular name, are rare.

The true Borderline Personality requires the most adept and mature of therapists and requires a commitment over a period of years of what is certain to be a stormy, difficult course.

Group Therapy

Group psychotherapy has proven of great value in the treatment of conditions in which denial is the primary mechanism of defense. This includes many of the Personality Disorders. To do proper group therapy requires a long period of training and great expertise. It may be unavailable in many areas.

The vast majority of people with Personality Disorders will never be treated for that specific condition. Perhaps the most important aspect of those who will work with them, in whatever role, is to be able to understand them sufficiently to gain their cooperation and, if possible, their respect. For example, if a man with a Paranoid Personality Disorder were hospitalized with traumatic injuries following an automobile accident, the most important thing might be to make the personality diagnosis and then to tailor the individual's treatment program for his injuries with that knowledge. The treatment of a similar patient with exactly the same injuries who had a Dependent Personality Disorder would be markedly different. Immediate closeness with a show of empathy would make the latter person feel secure whereas it would make the one with a Paranoid Personality Disorder frightened and anxious.

BIBLIOGRAPHY

Cleckley, H.: *The Mask of Sanity*. St. Louis, Mosby, 1955.

Cloninger, C.: The antisocial personality. *Hosp. Practice, 13:*96-106, 1978.

Kolb, L.: Personality Disorders. In *Modern Clinical Psychiatry,* pp. 603-628. Philadelphia, W.B. Saunders Co., 1977.

MacKinnon, R., and Michels, R.: The Hysterical Patient. In *The Psychiatric Interview in Clinical Practice,* pp. 110-146. Philadelphia, W.B. Saunders Co., 1971.

MacKinnon, R., and Michels, R.: The Paranoid Patient. In *The Psychiatric Interview in Clinical Practice,* pp. 259-295. Philadelphia, W.B. Saunders, Co., 1971.

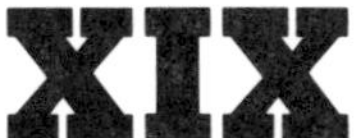

XIX

Treatment Modalities

Throughout this book the treatment of each diagnostic group has been mentioned briefly, with minimal description or explanation. This section will define the specific treatment modalities and their indications in more detail.

PSYCHOTHERAPY

There is no universally accepted definition of psychotherapy, but it often is referred to as the "talking cure." Most psychiatrists practice a form of psychotherapy known as "psychoanalytically oriented," meaning that it is based upon psychoanalytical theory, but is not classical psychoanalysis. There are innumerable variations and modifications but all more or less depend upon a thorough knowledge of the patient's background and personality, the development of a trusting relationship between the patient and the therapist, and the willingness and ability of the patient to express feelings and thoughts freely without fear of judgment or condemnation.

The psychotherapist must be able to be nonjudgmental and to be empathetic and understanding while tolerating the patient's attitudes and feelings even when they are negative and directed toward the therapist. This requires a thorough knowledge of one's own personality, a high level of maturity, and years of training and supervision.

Psychoanalysis

Psychoanalysis, the most intensive and probing type of psychotherapy, requires three or more hours per week, frequently for years, and is reserved for relatively well-adjusted people who wish to know more about themselves, people with classical neuroses, and for patients with other nonpsychotic illnesses. The time required, and the expense alone, limit this modality to a relatively small number of patients. Most psychiatrists are not trained fully in psychoanalysis–a discipline which requires years of study and controlled experience after the completion of formal psychiatric training.

Intensive Psychotherapy

This is based on the concepts of psychoanalysis, but has more limited goals. Sometimes called reconstructive, investigative, or insight psychotherapy, this modality aims to help the patient to achieve self-understanding, to clarify emotional conflicts, and to find a more effective way of dealing with the environment. It usually requires several months of from one to two hours weekly for a cooperative, well motivated patient. The factors at work in this type of psychotherapy are:

1. Uncovering and Abreaction

The recall of suppressed or repressed incidents and memories accompanied by the appropriate feeling and emotion is called abreaction.

2. Clarification and Reformulation

Incidents in the present life and in the past are related to the therapist who then can help the patient inspect and better understand the attitudes, feelings, and actions surrounding the event.

3. Desensitization

Uncovered incidents and events, once clarified, become less frightening and anxiety provoking and can be dealt with objectively.

4. Catharsis and Ventilation

Everyone knows that getting things "off the chest" makes one feel better, especially when done to a nonjudgmental, empathetic listener.

Supportive Psychotherapy

Supportive psychotherapy is a less intensive, more specifically aimed, and more goal-limited form of intensive psychotherapy. It may be needed to help a patient tolerate a period of crisis, or to help a patient with a chronic emotional problem to function as well as possible in the community in spite of the problem. It also should aim toward increasing self-esteem and self-confidence so that the patient may deal more effectively with the environment. The psychotherapy sessions more likely will be confined to the "here and the now," and uncovering and abreaction and catharsis will not be emphasized. It will be used briefly in many Adjustment Disorders, but may last for years in patients with Schizophrenia and other chronic disorders.

Group Psychotherapy

Certain conditions appear to respond better when from three to twelve patients meet with a therapist simultaneously. This type of psychotherapy may be indicated for patients whose difficulties involve relationship with peers, strong mechanisms of denial, or forms of acting-out behavior. This includes many of the sexual dysfunctions, especially the Paraphilias, types of Alcohol and Substance Abuse, many of the Personality Disorders, and Disorders of Impulse Control. Group psychotherapy is not merely a situation in which more people can be seen in a given amount of time. There should be positive indications for it, and many people feel that it is most effective when the members of the group have some problem in common.

BEHAVIORAL MODIFICATION

Behavioral modification implies that the behavior will be modified to relieve symptoms or to ameliorate problems, but that underlying emotional difficulties, if any, will not be involved. Most often it will be used for one specific symptom or act such as to relieve a simple phobia or to discourage Exhibitionism. Some of the therapeutic approaches of behavioral modification are:

1. Operant conditioning which consists of shaping behavior by having the patient do something that brings positive reinforcements for the desired behavior.
2. Desensitization has been used successfully in phobic patients by inducing relaxation, then systematically introducing the anxiety-provoking stimulus in a slowly increasing intensity. The patient may begin by imagining something resembling the phobic object then go through a series of steps including photographs or replicas until the object actually is touched.
3. Implosion is a method by which the patient is exposed to repeated horrifying accounts of, or contact with, a phobic object until desensitization takes place.
4. Aversive conditioning uses unpleasant stimuli, including pain, connected with undesirable behavior until that behavior is modified. For example, an alcoholic patient may be given his favorite drink which also contains a drug which makes him vomit. The homosexual male may be given an electric shock each time he gets an erection while looking at an attractive nude male.
5. Token economy is most popular on inpatient units or in institutional settings. Desirable behaviors are rewarded by giving the patient tokens which can be exchanged for privileges or objects that the patient desires. It is a form of operant conditioning.

There are many other aspects of behavioral modification, and many of them have yet to be accepted totally by Psychiatric Medicine. Some psychiatrists object to attempts to remove a single symptom without attending to the whole individual, but this, too, remains controversial.

SOMATIC TREATMENTS

Electroconvulsive Therapy (E.C.T.)

E.C.T. is a very effective treatment for severe depression. Deeply depressed patients with hallucinations and/or delusions do not respond well to any other form of treatment, therefore E.C.T.

is the treatment of choice. With modern techniques the patient does not convulse, has no pain, and no memory of the proceeding. The usual course is eight to twelve treatments given roughly every other day.

The exact method by which E.C.T. works is not know, but it appears to increase the level of the neurotransmitters that are believed to be deficient in the brain of depressed people. Approximately 90% of severely depressed people will respond favorably to E.C.T., and no other form of treatment has a success rate that high. Contrary to public opinion, E.C.T. is extremely safe, probably more so than any other form of treatment for severe depression, and there is no evidence that it produces brain damage. It is particularly indicated when the risk of suicide is great.

Medications

The most important medications used in Psychiatric Medicine are:

1. The antipsychotic drugs (major tranquilizers)
2. The antianxiety drugs (minor tranquilizers)
3. The antidepressants
4. Lithium carbonate

1. The Antipsychotic Drugs

This group of psychotropic drugs is especially effective in the treatment of psychotic symptoms. They appear to be beneficial by their ability to block dopamine receptors in the brain, especially in the limbic areas. Dopamine and its metabolites are the most important groups of neurotransmitters in the brain and particularly seem to be deranged in Schizophrenia and in the hypomanic and manic phases of Bipolar Disorder.

There are many forms of antipsychotic drugs, but the ones most commonly used are:

a. chlorpromazine (Thorazine)
b. thioridazine (Mellaril)
c. trifluoperazine (Stelazine)
d. fluphenazine (Prolixin and Permitil)

e. mesoridazine (Serentil)
f. haloperidol (Haldol)
g. thiothixene (Navane)
h. molindone hydrochloride (Moban)
i. loxapine (Loxitane)

There is no evidence that any one of these drugs is superior to the other when properly used in the correct dosage. The dosages vary considerably and, in general, the higher the milligrams per dose, the more sedating the drug. For example, Thorazine is much more sedating than Stelazine, and it takes 30 to 40 milligrams of Thorazine to equal one milligram of Stelazine. The choice of one drug over another might depend upon whether one wanted to produce sedation.

These drugs all have certain undesirable side effects. The most common are extrapyramidal syndromes and their variations. The term "extrapyramidal" refers to muscle dysfunctions which are not due to direct effect on the motor tracts in the brain, but come about through the indirect modulators of muscular activity in the basal ganglia. The syndromes include:

1. Akinesia which includes symptoms of muscle weakness, lethargy, and easy fatigability.
2. Akathisia which occurs in about 20% of the patients, more commonly in females. The most common symptom of akathisia is the inability to keep the legs still (restless legs syndrome).
3. Acute dystonia, more common in men and young patients, is a dramatic situation in which there is a severe spasm of muscles of the upper part of the trunk, neck, and/or face. The spasm of the neck muscle may produce extreme torticollis, or a spasm of some of the jaw muscles may freeze the mouth in an open, awkward position. Fortunately, the condition responds rapidly to certain drugs such as antihistamines and anticholinergics.
4. Parkinsonism, more common in women, usually occurs at higher doses of the antipsychotics. The patient may show all the signs of true Parkinsonism including a shuffling gait, a

mask-like face with increased salivation, generalized muscle rigidity, and a resting tremor of the hands. The condition responds well to anticholinergic medication, but sometimes will go away if the dose of the antipsychotic drug can be reduced.

5. Tardive Dyskinesia is the most serious of the major side effects. It occurs more frequently in elderly women who have been on an antipsychotic drug for a prolonged period of time, but is seen in younger patients and in men. The patient develops rhythmical involuntary movements of the face, mouth, jaw, and tongue. It may proceed to writhing, involuntary movements of the trunk and, in severe cases, the entire body. Unfortunately there is no known effective treatment for Tardive Dyskinesia. Discontinuing the drug, if at all possible, should be tried in the early phases, but all too frequently the patient then becomes overtly psychotic again.

   The symptoms will diminish if the drug dosage is increased, but gradully will return as the patient adjusts to the new level of medication. The only known method for preventing Tardive Dyskinesia is to keep the antipsychotic medication dose as low as possible and discontinue it as soon as possible. The medication cannot be discontinued or decreased in many cases of severe psychoses, so this condition remains one of great importance and presently is receiving tremendous amounts of research.

2. The Antianxiety Drugs (Minor Tranquilizers)

These drugs primarily are used to decrease anxiety, but also to induce sleep, to aid in seizure control (diazepam), and in the treatment of the withdrawal phase of some chemical dependency. They are more prone to abuse than are the major tranquilizers. Habituation can occur, and true addiction may be possible with large doses over a long period of time. They are safe, helpful drugs when used properly.

The minor tranquilizers work primarily in the limbic lobe of the brain and in the reticular activating system. They work by lowering neuron sensitivity by changes in the electrolytes in the synaptic areas. These drugs have little or no value in the psychoses and the major affective disorders. Some, especially chlordiazepoxide (Librium) and diazepam (Valium), may be used in the parenteral form in acute toxic brain syndromes, especially those due to withdrawal from alcohol (delirium tremens).

The antianxiety drugs include:

a. chlordiazepoxide (Librium)
b. diazepam (Valium)
c. oxazepam (Serax)
d. lorazepam (Ativan)
e. chlorazepate (Tranxene and Azene)
f. halazepam (Paxipam)
g. prazepam (Vestran)

There are many other drugs with antianxiety effects and new ones are coming on the market every few months. The antihistamines have calming potential, and meprobamate (Equanil and Miltown) and methaqualone (Quaalude) are effective, but the latter two are rarely used because they have a large habituation potential and no advantage over those listed.

Tolerance develops rather rapidly to most of the antianxiety drugs, and there appears to be a cross-tolerance with alcohol and many of the sedatives. They should be used in doses as low as possible for temporary relief of anxiety with few exceptions. One exception is the use of diazepam (Valium) as an adjunct to other treatments for some seizure disorders.

3. The Antidepressants

These drugs are most effective in Unipolar Depression and in the depressed phase of Bipolar Disorder. They act by making more neurotransmitters, primarily norepinephrine and serotonin, available in the synaptic clefts in the brain. Most of them require the full therapeutic dose from one to three weeks before becoming clinically effective. Those in common usage are:

a. imipramine (Tofranil)
b. desipramine (Pertofrane and Norpramin)

c. amitriptyline (Elavil and Endep)
d. nortriptyline (Aventyl)
e. doxepin (Sinequan and Adapin)
f. amoxapine (Asendin)
g. maprotiline (Ludiomil)
h. protriptyline (Vivactil)
i. phenelzine (Nardil)

The last drug, phenelzine, is a monoamine oxidase inhibitor (MAOI). It prevents or decreases the breakdown (oxidation) of monoamine (neurotransmitters) in the brain. This drug cannot be used without a specific diet which is relatlvey free of tyramine. It is indicated in certain milder forms of depression with a neurotic symptomatology, and requires that the patient be able to cooperate responsibly with the diet. Otherwise, there may be hypertensive crises and considerable danger of stroke and/or cardiac disease.

At least five new antidepressant drugs will be on the market by the time this book is published. Much research is directed toward these drugs because of the marked incidence of depression and because none of these drugs are 100% effective. Properly used in sufficient dose levels with the proper diagnosis they are, at best, 68% to 70% effective.

Other drugs have antidepressant properties, but only of a temporary nature. They include Dexedrine, Benzedrine, methylphenidate (Ritalin), and deanol. They have little clinical use because of their propensity to habituation and tolerance and the temporary nature of the relief they give the depressed patient. Methylphenidate has value in the treatment of some hyperactive children (Attention Deficit Disorder with Hyperactivity) and in a sleep disorder called Narcolepsy.

The main side effects of the antidepressant drugs are anticholinergic. They include dry mouth, exacerbation of glaucoma, blurred vision, orthostatic hypotension, cardiac arrhythmias, constipation, and urinary retention. Most of the side effects will respond to reducing the dose, if that is possible, but frequently the patient with a severe side effect will need to be changed to another form of antidepressant drug. A very undesirable side effect is that these drugs have become popular in suicide attempts.

Overdoses may be fatal, and since these drugs always are used in depressed patients, this possibility must be kept in mind. Patients and their families must be warned to keep the medication away from children.

4. *Lithium Carbonate*

Lithium carbonate is a drug of great value in the acute treatment and in the prevention of recurrences of the hypomanic and manic phases of Bipolar Disorder. The mechanism of action is thought to relate somehow to the exchange of sodium ions in the central nervous system, but is not known exactly. Patients who receive lithium must have an evaluation of the heart, liver, kidneys, and thyroid and, if these are normal, the drug is given four times daily, usually 300 milligrams or more per dose, until a blood level of 0.8 to 1.5 millequivalents per liter (meq/L) is attained. The antimanic effect usually takes five to eight days and, during this period of waiting, it may be necessary to use large doses of one of the antipsychotic medications.

Once the patient is stabilized, serum lithium levels can be measured every one to three months with safety. The drug appears to have a major prophylactic effect against recurrent manic and hypomanic attacks, but may not be so effective in preventing the depressive phases of the illness. The antidepressants can be used effectively with lithium if the patient becomes depressed after the manic phase.

The toxic effects of lithium indicate a serum lithium level probably over 1.8 meq/L. The symptoms are nausea, vomiting, diarrhea, lethargy, mental confusion, thirst, and a fine tremor which is worse in the hands. Unless the blood level is reduced, the syndrome can progress to coma, convulsions, and death in two or three days. Toxic blood levels can occur if the patient perspires too much in very hot weather or has episodes of diarrhea and/or uses a low salt or salt free diet. Hypothyroidism can occur, and it is good to check thyroid function and renal clearance at least annually. There is some evidence that the long-term use may produce some renal damage, but this slight danger must be balanced against the need for the medication. Many people may need to be on the drug for years, even for life, depending upon the severity of their Bipolar Disorder and the frequency with which they have the episodes. Lithium is the only drug in Psychiatric Medicine with a true preventive potential.

Psychopharmacology is a fast growing, ever changing field. Knowledge of the brain's neurochemistry is increasing more than any other aspect of medicine so that exciting advances in the treatment of mental illness can be expected in the near future.

BIBLIOGRAPHY

Abse, W.: *Clinical Notes on Group-Analytic Psychotherapy.* Charlottesville, The U. of Virginia Press, 1974.

Adler, M.: Psychoanalysis and psychotherapy. *Int. J. Psychoanalysis, 51:*219, 1970.

Behavior Therapy in Psychiatry, Task Force Report of the American Psychiatric Association. New York, Jason Aronson, 1974.

Colby, K.: *A Primer for Psychotherapists.* New York, Roland Press, 1951.

Dunner, D., Stollone, F., and Fieve, R.: Lithium carbonate and affective disorders. *Arch. Gen. Psychiatry, 33:*117, 1976.

Hollister, L.: Use of psychotherapeutic drugs. *Ann. Intern. Med., 79:*88, 1973.

Kessler, K., and Waletzky, J.: Clinical use of antipsychotics. *Am. J. Psychiatry, 138:*202, 1981.

Liberman, R. (ed.): Behavioral Therapy in Psychiatry. In *Psychiatric Clin. North Am., 1:*2. Philadelphia, W.B. Saunders Co., 1978.

Simpson, S. (ed.): *Drug Treatment of Mental Disorders.* New York, Raven Press, 1976.

Index